Cheers to Queers

Stories of Coming Out,
Finding Community
and Saving My Life

by
Moushumi Ghose

Moons Grove Press
British Columbia, Canada

Cheers to Queers:
Stories of Coming Out, Finding Community and Saving My Life

Copyright ©2025 by Moushumi Ghose
ISBN-13 978-1-77143-605-2
First Edition

Library and Archives Canada Cataloguing in Publication
Title: Cheers to queers : stories of coming out, finding community and saving my life /
by Moushumi Ghose.
Names: Ghose, Moushumi, 1972- author.
Identifiers: Canadiana (print) 20240339665 | Canadiana (ebook) 20240339746
| ISBN 9781771436052 (softcover) | ISBN 9781771436069 (PDF)
Subjects: LCSH: Ghose, Moushumi. | LCSH: Bisexual women—United States—Biography.
| LCSH: Bisexual people—United States—Biography.
| LCSH: Bengali American women—Biography.
| LCSH: Bengali Americans—Biography. | LCSH: Bisexual people—Identity.
| LCGFT: Autobiographies.
Classification: LCC HQ74.43.G46 A3 2024 | DDC 306.76/50820973—dc23

Artwork credit: Front cover artwork © Lisa Truong, used with permission.

Moons Grove Press is an imprint
of CCB Publishing: www.ccbpublishing.com

Moons Grove Press
British Columbia, Canada
www.moonsgrovepress.com

Dedicated to all those who struggle with identity.
May you find your voice and a world that accepts you.

Contents

INTRODUCTION

Keep Smiling Even When Your Heart Is in A Million Pieces (and other thoughts)

The essays in this collection chronicle how the LGBTQ community would be the light that shined and showed me the way in the 1980's.

But it wasn't always easy.

I was hanging out with the queers, the lesbians, the gays, the misfits, the oppressed. Yes, my friend groups, which consisted of Asian, Black, and Latino was growing. I was grateful to live in such multi-cultural places.

At home, a quiet suburb about 26 miles east of San Francisco, my family was a part of a big Bengali (from eastern India) community (our chosen family in the US), which was small in the 1970's and has now grown to be quite substantial. Growing up, I would spend weekends with our Bengali friends. These families had many Bengali kids my age. These people felt like our own family because like my parents, they had immigrated from India, spoke the language, understood the culture and were all having similar experiences, working, living and raising families here in the US.

But, I lived in two worlds.

Back at school my friends were distinctly American. Everyone spoke English. Cross culture mingling was frowned upon. In school, we were expected to assimilate. I had a different set of friends at school than the families and kids I would spend time with on the weekends. As I got older this would change... very slowly.

I once read this article in *Time Magazine* about the difference between Indian immigrants and other minority groups. The question was: Why weren't there predominantly Indian parts of town, like Chinatown, or predominantly Black and Latino neighborhoods? The reason the article gave was assimilation. Indian people were more likely to assimilate into integrated neighborhoods than to stay in their own neighborhoods.

I resonated with that article. My entire experience resonated with that article. We had always assimilated, and on weekends we found our people. All of whom were also assimilating.

Being a person of color in the United States is a complicated story, and I'm trying to untangle it.

One of my teenage club friends turned into a lifelong trauma bond.[1] A trauma bond is a complex connection which has elements of abuse, such as manipulation, gaslighting, exploitation and other forms of control that often creeps in after the victim is deeply invested.

I remember when she came to my hometown, she asked me with disdain in her voice, "Is this an Indian neighborhood?"

---

[1] For a definition of Trauma Bond refer to the following article: https://www.oprahdaily.com/life/relationships-love/a36788688/what-is-trauma-bonding

I felt defensive. I was embarrassed that she would consider me to be anything but American. Now I struggle with the opposite. I find myself angry when people act like they don't see my color. "I am Indian, you know." My perfect American English dialect leaves my American friends thinking my experience was like theirs. Which it wasn't. And the real trigger is that I am afraid I am losing connection to my Indian roots. I am upset that they don't see it. Or that they forget.

The same friend also asked me once, "Where are all your Indian friends?" I am confused. What is the message here? Do you or don't you want me to surround myself with Indian people? Should I or shouldn't I be proud of my heritage?

All the mixed messaging turned me into one giant people pleaser, traumatized to my core. And, well that was the point, wasn't it? To confuse the fuck out of me, to disarm me and basically emotionally maim and paralyze me. And, well it worked (at least, temporarily) and would've really done a number on me, if I didn't know better, and didn't want more for myself. And it took me a really long time to unlearn these stories. And, sometimes I think that in the 1980's and 1990's people just talked that way. Rude. Degrading. Sarcastic. That's what this book is about. Most of the messaging I received was of the disabling sort. People weren't very nice. And I learned the hard way. And, I wanted better. I was seeking better. But, in the process, I had to give up a lot. My journey is that of getting back what I lost.

For South Asian Indians, assimilating is seen as a simultaneously good and bad thing. People of color cannot win. The hardest part is that you must just keep smiling. Keep your head up and keep smiling even though in your heart you are breaking into a million pieces.

* * *

Before read this, I'd like to share a few words I use throughout the book, and to give you my definitions for them to clear up any confusion before you even get there.

These words have become political in nature, and that has made them highly controversial, loaded, and a hotbed for discourse. Mainly people don't *really truly* understand the meaning behind the words and therefore take them personally. I want to assure you, they are not personally targeted at any person, gender, race. *They are used in context of a much larger system, a macrosystem (of global culture) that we are all a part of.*

This book is about a complicated coming of age journey, but I can't untangle that from my experiences as a brown, American born, child of immigrants. So it's all a big mash up and I am just trying to deliver in a way that's somehow easy to digest. With that said, here are some of those terms:

- Toxic Masculinity – This is a huge one. So many men think this is about them. ***This is not about men.*** I have (created or produced) a lot of videos and continue to spend time and energy educating on this topic. This is about the culture we live in that prides masculine behavior and assigns masculine behavior to males. It encourages men to act a certain, extreme way, and for women to act in a complementary way. It is in fact extremely binary which doesn't leave room for the rest of us, which is read: most of us.

Here is how Toxic Masculinity is defined in Wikipedia[2]:

Toxic masculinity is a set of certain male behaviors associated with harm to society and men themselves. Stereotypical aspects of traditional masculinity, such as social dominance, misogyny, and homophobia, can be considered "toxic" due in part to their promotion of

---

[2] Source: https://en.wikipedia.org/wiki/Toxic_masculinity

violence, including sexual assault and domestic violence. Socialization of boys often normalizes violence, such as in the saying "boys will be boys" about bullying and aggression.

Self-reliance and emotional repression are correlated with increased psychological problems in men such as depression, increased stress, and substance use disorders. Toxic masculine traits are characteristic of the unspoken code of behavior among men in prisons, where they exist in part as a response to the harsh conditions of prison life.

Other traditionally masculine traits such as devotion to work, pride in excelling at sports, and providing for one's family, are not considered to be "toxic." The concept was originally used by authors associated with the mythopoetic men's movement, such as Shepherd Bliss. These authors contrasted stereotypical notions of masculinity with a "real" or "deep" masculinity, which they said men had lost touch with in modern society. Critics of the term toxic masculinity argue that it incorrectly implies that gender-related issues are caused by inherent male traits.

The concept of toxic masculinity, or certain formulations of it, has been criticized by some conservatives as an undue condemnation of traditional masculinity, and by some feminists as an essentialist concept that ignores the role of choice and context in causing harmful behaviors and attitudes related to masculinity.

It is important to acknowledge that toxic masculinity is the same side of toxic femininity, they complement each other, and exist together because of each other. They exist in tandem within a patriarchy.

I use toxic masculinity interchangeably with terms like "straight poop" (a word my friend discovered on a bumper sticker at the Castro Street train station in San Francisco), heteronormative, and homophobia, as they all tend to converge on the same side of the plate. Many sides to one coin. You see, we are taught very narrow, binary forms of gender and sexual expression from a very young age. We are conditioned to see, for example, couples of the opposite gender getting married and mating long-term. This is the "normative." This is not to say that this is normal. In fact, the continuum of human nature and human sexuality is much greater than what we have been conditioned to do and see. Much of these expressions, which lay outside the "normative," have been invisible and erased. When we see something that is outside of the "normative," we assume that it is not normal. But it is. We judge it harshly because we are unfamiliar with those expressions that are on the fringe, like homophobia, transphobia, and the likes. Therefore the "normative" view while being the prevalent view and also continuously perpetuated in every facet of our culture via media, television, and corporations, is problematic, and the people who do not see this problem are often the ones who end up causing more harm.

- Sex Positive – It is defined by Allena Gabosch as: "An attitude towards human sexuality that regards all consensual sexual activities as fundamentally healthy and pleasurable, encouraging sexual pleasure and experimentation."[3] The sex positive movement also advocates for comprehensive sex education and safe sex as part of its campaign.

- Feminism – Usually I will be referring to third-wave of feminism.

---

[3] Source: Allena Gabosch:
https://allenagabosch.wordpress.com/2014/12/08/a-sex-positive-renaissance - Used with permission.

In 1992 Rebecca Walker, a 23-year-old Black bisexual woman, first used the term third-wave feminism. Third-wave feminism became more conscious of race. While the first- and second-wave of feminism had ignored or neglected racial disparities within gender, the third-wave paid more attention.

And, as of late, the consensus is changing. Again. I just heard on a podcast this morning that Feminism was created by the patriarchy to support capitalism. I buy it, and also don't have time to dwell on this anymore.

- Fluid – I identify as Bi and Fluid. I use the words interchangeably. To me, coming of age in the 1980s, "bisexual" was an all-encompassing term. Today some people prefer "pansexual" to "bisexual," to identify a person who is attracted to a person regardless of gender. "Pansexual" is more inclusive as there are more than two genders.

However, the definition of Bisexual is a person who is sexually attracted not exclusively to people of one particular gender.

- White Supremacy and White Privilege – White Supremacy is generally accepted as an institutionally perpetuated system of exploitation and oppression of continents, nations, and peoples of color by white peoples and nations of the European continent. The purpose is to maintain and defend a system of wealth, power, and privilege. As a system, racism affects every aspect of life in a country. White Supremacy has been more useful than the term racism because "supremacy" defines a power relationship.

***Note: I want to mention that the stories included here happened many years ago. Most of these people in the stories were mere children, young. Everyone was trying their best with the tools they were given. These stories are not to point fingers or to place blame. They are my stories, my experiences and what I felt I had to overcome to heal myself and get to where I am today.

The Truth Is
BY MOUSHUMI GHOSE

The truth is I did something for someone else
That I didn't care to do
To feel safe

The truth is I didn't believe in myself
To be real

The truth is I could have been something else
Done something else for a much harder means

The truth is I misplaced my youth
If you were to ask me

But there is the other story
That this was all somehow meant to be

The truth is
Most likely
That this is all meant to be

໒ Chapter 1 ໒

Rat's Nest Barbie
1979

Guilty as charged. I played with Barbie as a young girl. This is hard to admit as a brown person who detests traditional gender roles. Over the years Barbie has gone under a lot of scrutiny for perpetuating an ideal for girls and women that is unattainable. Today, Barbie comes in all colors, and many more shapes and sizes in an attempt to become more inclusive. When I played with Barbie, they all had blonde hair and white skin. In those days, she drove a pink corvette. The Barbie saga is one that has plagued many children because of its reach and its power to model one very specific way of being as the normative. She was skinny, blonde, lacking in genitals and had only the feminine characteristics of a female, which meant wearing pink, the color used to refer to girls, the female gender. Children got to decide, in their play, what type of woman Barbie would be. In the 1970s Barbie was a trophy wife or girlfriend. Today, Barbie goes to work and has a variety of skin colors, due to the outrage that many social justice groups have been vocal about. Barbie has become a symbol of feminism and inclusivity. But it wasn't always like that.

The year Beauty Secrets Barbie came out, it was all the rage. She had long thick hair, down to her butt. Me and my gal pals all had to have Beauty Secrets Barbie. I was in the third grade.

* * *

But, first I should talk about skin color, if I am to talk about Barbie.

I can't really recall when I became aware of my skin color. I must have been around 5 or 6, when I first experienced what we now know today as White Supremacy (see definition in the Introduction).

We had just moved into our new home, a home that I've come to consider my childhood home. My sister was just a newborn, and we moved into a brand spanking new tract housing development in a small agricultural suburb about 26 miles east of San Francisco, California. The town was called Walnut Creek. This day all the neighbors were getting together to plan the fence building.

One of the other families had a young, blonde-haired, blue-eyed daughter my age. Julee. I smiled at her, excited to see another girl my age, eager to make new friends. Immediately, without flinching or doing a double take, and instead of smiling back, she stuck her tongue out at me with a scowl on her face that would send the strongest of lions back to their den, tail between their legs. My heart sank. I felt my stomach drop, I know that feeling now was one of deep fear, and then sadness. My soul recoiled at such hostility. This is my first memory of true hostility. Children learn from their parents. Julee's father was rude to me, my mother, and probably to my father too, although I never asked my parents. I always felt these subtle jabs were because we were so obviously different from them, with our darker skin color, our foreign accents, the food we ate which was drenched in spices like curry and coriander, and the way we dressed. How I wanted to fit in, to be accepted by Julee.

Julee and I would become friends, though. Which is really more to say we played and spent a lot of time together. Friends may be a little too strong of a word, as I don't think Julee ever really liked me. Although it was all I ever really wanted.

Julee was very popular at school, especially with the boys, and later with the girls. She was always picked first for kickball. I was usually picked last, even though I could out run everyone. If young girls can be hot, Julee was it. Of course, as her close friend, I felt like the ugly duckling.

I was more like a sidekick, a little puppy that followed along, rather than a true friend.

Julee and I had a third friend, Fiona. Fiona was sweet from day one. Kind. Her parents were kind people also. The three of us often had playdates after school. Like most of the kids at my school she also had blonde hair and blue eyes. Fiona always welcomed me with open arms, and I appreciated her for it. Her family was also very kind and inclusive. Were Fiona and I friends? I always wanted to believe so, but when you are kind to everyone I couldn't help but wonder what she thought of me underneath, what her ears would hear when I wasn't around. But, still, at least she always led with kindness.

Excitedly we all introduced Beauty Secrets Barbie to our play. She stood out from all our previous Barbies because of her hair, one, which I mentioned was long and thick, straight down past her butt, but also because she was new, different from all the other Barbies. Little 6-year-old me never gave much thought to the fact that Barbie didn't share my skin color. In fact, Barbie's skin was tanned, so it felt somewhat close to mine. But, the hair was clearly blonde. Besides our skin and hair color, however, something was amiss with my Beauty Secrets Barbie. When she came out of the box her hair was fine, long, and brush-able, but at some point, something happened. I woke up to find that Beauty Secret Barbie's hair looked like a wild rat's nest.

I tried to comb it, but the smoothness and shine was gone from my beloved Barbie's hair. I put her hair in a ponytail and put her in my bag. I would deal with it later. I was more worried that my friends would notice.

Sure enough, Fiona saw it first and asked, "What's going on with your Barbie's hair?"

I looked away and kept playing. I had really hoped it wasn't that visible.

Julee, of course, upon hearing Fiona's statement, turned right around and gawked.

"OH MY GOD WHAT IS WRONG WITH YOUR BARBIE'S HAIR?" She said it so loud. Julee loved to point at and embarrass people.

Now, both of their eyes were on my Barbie. It was obvious. And out there.

Ashamed, I shrugged and said, "I just need to wet it and brush it."

Mouths gaping wide, both were aghast. "Your poor Barbie." As if I had done something terribly wrong.

But the symbolism of my Barbie's hair was not lost on me. Even their Barbies had better hair than mine. And I couldn't do anything right.

Yes, the symbolism I am referring to is my own head of hair. Indian girl hair. It's thick, it's black, it's wavy, sometimes curly, and frizzy. I did not know how to manage my hair. My mother didn't either. She was an immigrant from India, and the rules for hairstyles in India were far different from the hairstyles of the west. For one, in the US, wearing our hair down is normal. In India, in the late 1950s and 1960s when she was growing up, wearing your hair down was a sign of tawdriness and considered disrespectful. It suggested that you were loose, easy perhaps. So, thick wavy-haired me, who really could've benefited from long hair, because I would learn much later that longer hair supports curls and waves, by weighing the curls down making them less poufy and giving the curls more definition. Nope, instead, I was to wear my hair shoulder length – all of my childhood.

In this day and age, with all the hair tools, serums and potions available to us, short hair is doable for a curly, wavy, coarse-haired girl like myself, but for a little Indian girl, growing up in suburban America in the 1970s whose mother knew nothing of hair dryers or curling irons, my cowlicks and curls were chopped and brushed out which did not suit my unruly hair.

In India, then, they also did a few other things Westerners would find odd. Not sure these traditions still hold up, but I'm sure they do in some parts. They used oil, coconut oil instead of shampoo. While this is actually really great for your hair in between washes particularly for my thick curly-haired compatriots, it does not support western beauty standards of silky, shiny smooth hair.

The oily look, which led to dandruff because of the lack of shampoo allowing all the dirt on the scalp to collect and shine bright on my oily slick greasy black hair, did not do my popularity in grade school, in the American suburbs, any favors. In fact, I was the laughingstock of the class.

By the time I reached the third grade, my mother had grown tired of fighting with me to brush my hair. Frankly, it hurt like hell when she would try to comb it out. Like my Barbie I, too, often donned a rat's nest.

I stood out like a sore thumb.

That night I tried everything to make Beauty Secrets Barbie's hair smooth again. I used water, shampoo, conditioner. I combed it, put it in a braid and let it dry overnight. I was determined to fix her hair and get it back to the way it was. It had too, right? I mean, it had come out of the box that way. And, I must have done something to make her hair look so ratty.

When I woke up, I went and checked on Barbie. I carefully unbraided her hair, which was still wet and tried to comb it through. Nothing. It was still as ratty as before, maybe even more so.

What was I going to do? I couldn't show up again with rat's hair nest Barbie. I had to get a new Barbie, however there was no way my parents would buy me another one. They were strict about buying too many toys. But, I had to prove to Fiona and Julee that I could be good. That I was good enough.

And, then I had an idea.

That afternoon before we headed out to go to the grocery store, I ran to my room and took Beauty Secrets Barbie's head off the doll and shoved it down my pants. It was worth a shot.

Once we got to the store, I told my mom I was going to the toy section.

"I will be right back."

"Don't go too far," my mom yelled back.

I had to be quick. I b-lined to the Barbie section and found the rows of Barbies. I looked up and around and finally there she was, beautifully packaged in the silky pink box, and untouched, a perfectly manicured, soft-flowing-haired, new Beauty Secrets Barbie. She glowed!

I quickly opened the box and opened up the packaging, and snapped the head off of the brand new Barbie doll, and touched her smooth hair. Ah yes, this was perfect. A momentary rush came over me at the thought that I was going to have a soft-haired Barbie once again. I then took the old rat's nest head out and shoved it into the box, haphazardly, and fumbled as I tried to shut the box and get out of there as quickly as I could. I needed to get back to my parents before they started looking for me. I put the new head down my pants, and ran back to meet my parents.

"Where did you go?" my mom asked.

"Oh, I just went to see something in the toy section."

The next time I was at Fiona's, she noticed right away. "How did you fix her hair?" she asked suspiciously.

"Oh, I just shampooed it and it got better," I said casually and went back to playing with the dolls.

"Really?" She did not look satisfied with my answer. Her eyes said to me, "I know you stole that head." But she did not say anything else.

"Yes, I know, how cool, right?"

And we never spoke of it again. In fact, after that day we barely played with Beauty Secrets Barbie ever again.

❧ Chapter 2 ❧

The Oak Ridge Girls
1981

I was 9 when we moved to Oak Ridge, Tennessee for two years. My dad was going to work at a lab there. I didn't want to leave my friends. I didn't want to go to a new school. We rented out our house in California. We were coming back.

Oak Ridge was a different world. It was green, there are lots of trees and forest everywhere and the people were insanely nice. We lived in a big house that had a giant yard and a long spiraling driveway. It looked so different to the dry desert-like suburb of California where I came from.

And, it snowed in Oak Ridge. Not a lot, but enough to go tobogganing in the winter.

I had never experienced such niceness in my life. It was the fourth grade and I immediately made friends and I was popular with my peers. People wondered if my brown skin was because I was from California. My teacher, Mrs. Stevens, asked me if I spoke English. I think she was surprised to see that I spoke it very well. I told her I was born in the United States and that I was living in California. There weren't many South Asians in the US, let alone the south, at the time.

Like I said, everyone was so nice with the exception of Latoya Jones, who made it known that she didn't like me.

And she also made it known that she wanted to fight me. Me? What did I do. It was the first time I would experience fighting in school, like real physical fighting among girls in my life. Should I be scared? I kind of laughed it off. The next thing you know Latoya and her crew came up to me. They were letting me know that it was time to fight. I really don't remember what happened next, but I used all my strength and I bent Latoya's arm around. She was smaller than me, she was thinner than me, and I found out she was also weaker than me. And all of a sudden, she let go. She must have known this was pointless. I wasn't prepared to fight, but I guess I would if I had to.

Instead, she laughed and said, "Just kidding," and the next thing you know we were friends.

LaToya hung around another gal, Lisa. Suddenly Lisa and Latoya would come over to where I was sitting at lunch and sit with me. It was almost like I had been jumped into a gang. But we were nothing like a gang. We talked about music and make-up. We had sleepovers and watched movies.

And, for two years, during 4th and 5th grades, I had these girls as my best friends. We were a multicultural gang of girls. There were eight of us. We were a group of Asian, black, Caucasian and Hispanic. And we wore our skin color with pride. One of the girls was immediately my friend because our fathers worked together at the lab. She was also from California. And, slowly our group grew. I'm not even sure how it happened. There was Lisa and Latoya. There was Margaret and Nell. We were inseparable. There was always someone to talk to and hang out with at lunch, at assembly. It was a fun time, and I had never met a group of girls who were so nice.

But it was short lived. After two years my family was slated to move back to California.

I was personally excited to go back. I was excited to see my old friends and to share with them everything I had learned and experienced in this other place: the south. I guess I never committed to calling it home.

It was late summer as we finally pulled up into our old garage in that California suburb. My Dad parked the car and we all got out.

I saw my old friend Julee riding by on her bike.

Seeing us, she stopped and asked, "You're back?" She was expressionless.

"Hi," my family all cheered. Everyone was happy to see her. My mom, dad, sister and of course me.

"Yes, we only went for two years," I said eagerly.

"Oh, cool," she said, warming up a little. "Will you be at school?"

"Yes, I will be there!" I exclaimed excitedly. I was looking forward to seeing all my friends again.

"See you there," Julee said nonchalantly as she rode off.

Julee hadn't been too excited to see me, but I was still hopeful. The first day of 6th grade, I saw my old school friends all hanging out in a circle. I walked over, looking forward to talking to everyone. But no one said hi, no one parted ways to include me in the circle. I just stood there on the outside of the circle. Me and another brown Hispanic girl who was also hanging around. And Julee, she was in the center. The main attraction. And everyone clamoring to be her friend.

I suddenly realized I didn't fit in here. Maybe I never had. My old friends had changed and didn't recognize me anymore. I didn't recognize them. I went from having a tight knit group of diverse girlfriends to being alone and outcast at a school where everyone looked the same and dressed the same. I wasn't small, blonde, nor blue eyed. I was even laughed at because I had bad style, a funny hairdo, and mostly I was just an awkward and gawky pre-teen who had grown tall before everyone else. And no one seemed to care about having me around.

I spent the rest of the year lonely, sad, and anxious. I was desperate to fit in.

I looked forward to 7th grade, Junior High, and all but forgot about Oak Ridge and my time there.

❧ Chapter 3 ❧

English Soap
1983

Oh, American girl
Look in the mirror
You look ravishing in your leather skirt
So do you my dear
Said the Brit, as she smacked her shiny red lips
BY MOUSHUMI GHOSE

I was an awkward 11-year-old that summer, just starting to wake up from my little girl haze of childhood into the pubescent consciousness of my adolescence. When we arrived in London, it was hot and sweaty in late July and there was a reservation mix-up at our hotel. My dad, mom, my sister and I, plus another couple and their small child, descended upon the last place remaining to spend the night at a youth hostel.

My father, who was typically so organized, hadn't been able to book us a room at a regular hotel as he typically would, something that was family friendly. To their liking. But for whatever reason tonight the city was completely booked, with the exception of this youth hostel where we had to suck it up for one night, sharing a bathroom with the entire floor. We were only in London for one night anyway. In the morning, we were heading to France, via Ferry, across the English Channel, where we would rent a car to drive across the rest of Europe for a summer vacation.

This wasn't the first time I had traveled overseas. My family and I traveled a lot back and forth to India, allowing us many layovers which led my dad, a geographic genius, among other things, to split up our trips to include many stops in many countries. I consider myself lucky.

But despite traveling a lot, I had been sheltered. I had known but one existence: the world through my parent's eyes. Children are mostly sponges – molded into humans by our parent's hand, or whoever raises us. Our caregivers. They shape us in so many ways. Growing up in the US, my mother would over-prepare us for India whenever we traveled there. She'd say, "We must pack toilet paper," and, "Don't drink the water." Not to mention all the shots we had to get to protect our immune systems from the shock. We grew up with a fear of India being dangerous to our health. My father, on the other hand, would use geographic facts to sometimes make dad jokes: "Today we're going to see the giant arch in St Louis, it's like the McDonald's arch but not as gold," or, "Did you know that Oklahoma is just OK?" Hahaha, very funny, Dad.

But, this trip was different. I don't know if it was because I was older, or I was seeing something like Europe for the first time, which is quite different for Americans. Was it the architecture of the buildings, which are older and classical? Was it the quaintness of the streets which were often narrow with cobblestones? Or was it my age, the spritely young age of 11 when you start changing? This trip was different because, this time, I definitely noticed everything.

En route to the hostel in London we encountered lots of street folk, including an old homeless woman angrily mumbling to herself.

Finally, after what seemed like many hours on the phone and en route in a taxi, we arrived and checked into the old Victorian era hostel in what felt like downtown London. The building was about 4 stories high and shaped like a box, with pillars of lions out front. The bedroom was just a room with gray, drab, gothic style wallpaper that was faded and looked like it had been there for years. There were two full-sized beds and a sink. A sink? In the bedroom? I had never seen such a thing.

The bathroom was down the long hall, which had the same style wallpaper, stained and old. The bathroom was shared with others who lived on the floor.

I sheepishly walked down the long scary hall by myself to use the bathroom. It was an old bathroom with several stalls. I found my way into the stall and felt a rush of fear as I used the seemingly ancient toilet with its flush that hung from the ceiling. I always hated bathrooms, especially the ones in other countries. As an American child, everywhere else in the world seems old, and bathrooms are always where you notice the antiquity first.

I finished my business and came out of the stall. As I washed my hands and planned to leave the bathroom in a hurry, I was overcome by a sense of something else, something new, something fresh and alive. For the first time, I saw a world different than anything I had ever experienced in my whole life of 11 years, in my microcosm. It was like I had finally stepped out into another world. Suddenly, I saw a whole new macrocosm, full of color, diversity, hope, and intrigue. For the first time, I think I saw a future for me.

There were two women.

The two women in the bathroom were getting ready to go out, a night on the town. Black stilettos, leather pants, red lipstick and short skirts. The blonde girl had an American accent, in her gray off-the-shoulder top and white mini skirt.

A black-haired British woman in black, shiny, patent leather pants with a black off-the-shoulder top was talking. She had on red lipstick and big earrings. They were standing in front of the mirrors.

"Oh, you are going to love it here." The British woman said to the American woman. "Your outfit is perfect."

The American woman stood next to her, watching her apply her lipstick. "Really? I think *you* look amazing. I just love your hair."

"Here you go, use this." The British woman handed the American woman her lipstick.

"You think it's too much?" The American girl applied the bright red lipstick and was admiring herself in the mirror.

"No, not at all. You look amazing." Then she continued, "Oh, you are going to love this club. The music is great, and we can go until 4 AM. Plus, I am super excited for you to meet Roe." The British woman smoothed her hair as her bracelets jingled. She was no nonsense.

The American woman, clearly visiting London, a guest, and excited at that moment, flipped her head back, laughed and said, "Great, let's go then!"

As I dried my hands, I lingered. I wanted to hear more. But the blonde finished applying her lipstick and then the two turned around and hurriedly walked out the door, laughing and talking all the while.

Their bracelets jingled and their high heels clicked on the tile as they left the bathroom. The smell of British soap and French perfume hung in the air. My world had been flipped on its side. There was suddenly a portal to another world, something mysterious and exciting, colorful and dangerous. I wanted to walk through it.

I hung back for a bit, before leaving and catching a glimpse of my drab American suburban child's clothes in the mirror. At least I could dream.

"Mind the Gap." It's what the voice on the speaker says when you ride the London Underground. The humidity hung in the air. I sat down with my parents in a trance as I watched the fabulous circus unfold in front of my eyes: pink mohawks, boys in black eyeliner, studded leather jackets, giant safety pins, black jazz shoes with laces, fishnet stockings, frilly blouses, red leather gloves. I was entranced. This was the center of the world, as far as I was concerned. London 1983. Never had I seen so much color and electricity.

We traveled around Europe that summer, and the entire trip I was knee-deep in my imagination. In my daydream, I was older, a woman. I was stylish. I had lovers and intrigue. In reality, I was an awkward pre-pubescent girl.

We had one more stop in London. As we walked the hot and sweltering streets in the August heat, I noticed an older homeless woman with pale skin and jet-black hair. I had seen her the last time I was there. She was walking in the crosswalk, angrily mumbling to herself. I immediately felt a familiarity.

In the air hung the scent of British soap, a scent I remembered from that day in the bathroom from last time I was there. A scent that is forever emblazoned in my memory. The smell will forever remind me of London, England in 1983, and what I had experienced. I was changed forever. I had seen something I could never unsee. I was awakened. And, I would hang onto the memory until I would find it, a place in the world like this for me to fit in.

❧ Chapter 4 ☙

Trying Way Too Hard
1984-1985

I remember what I wore the day we toured around Tokyo. I was 13 and falling in love with the fashion of the times. I had on a wool houndstooth pencil skirt that had 3 pleats in the front and landed around my calves. I wore lace-up black flats and my dad's oversized wool sweater. I really should have worn socks or something warmer on my feet. December in Tokyo was cold.

There were only a few people at my school who seemingly had similar taste and style. But they were not people I was close friends with.

Hailey and Dolan. Both wore all black, black eyeliner and had black hair. And, more recently they had started talking to me. They were part of the cool kids.

"Are you leaving?" Hailey said out of the blue, passing me in the hallway.

"I'm going to Asia for a month."

"Oh, really?" Dolan exclaimed.

"Wow, that's cool," Hailey said in a lower tone.

I didn't say much more and parted ways with them, but I was feeling very good about our interaction. I felt seen by two kids who were part of a bigger popular crowd who had for some reason taken an interest in me in recent weeks. I wasn't sure why they were talking to me, but I was excited to see where this would go. Could it be my fabulously forward sense of style or was it my great taste in music? I was gushing.

But it was true. I was leaving in a few days for a month-long trip to Asia. People at school knew, because I had to miss one month of school which was kind of a big deal. And, that also meant, I was not going to be able to see this new friendship through. It would have to wait.

We hadn't been to India in several years. In fact, the last time I had gone I was 5 or 6 years old. A small child. Now a pre-teen I was looking more and more adult every day. Or so I thought. I was naïve and still had so much to learn.

My dad took us everywhere. A trip to India meant, how many other cities, both in India and in other countries, can we squeeze in along the way? Evidently, it was many. Tokyo and Hong Kong were spots we were going to hit on this trip. On another trip around we would hit Kuala Lumpur, Singapore, Bangkok all en route to our main stop, which was always Calcutta, India. (Now it's called Kolkata, India – which is the Indian spelling and pronunciation. Post-colonial India began to reclaim the original city names once British occupation ended in 1947. It has taken over 50 years for these original names to stick.)

Calcutta /Kolkata is where my parents are both from and where all my extended family and my relatives all lived when I was a child. We had no other family in the United States. (As I write this people have dispersed. Some of the younger generation have come to the States, or relocated to other cities in India, Canada, UK and more.) During that time of my childhood, we created what is known as "chosen family." We became close with so many other Bengali immigrants who lived in the Bay Area. They became our extended families.

I was falling in love with the world and I was learning that outside my little suburb, there was more. Much more.

In the streets of Tokyo, I bought the cutest little, tiniest Sony Walkman I had ever seen. It was shiny, silver, and barely the size of a tape cassette. It was sleek and the cassette just slid out of the casing which opened and closed on its own, without so much as a button. I loved this high-tech stylish Walkman that I had never seen in the United States. Of course, the entire manual was written in Japanese, and so when it stopped working a few months later after we were back in the US, it was not repairable. This was life back then. Today we might find a Japanese speaking person, but that wasn't the way things worked then. Still, I cherished that Walkman and kept it for many years.

In the streets of Hong Kong, which was independent in 1984, I was mesmerized by the styles. (Today Hong Kong belongs to China and was delivered from the United Kingdom to the People's Republic of China at midnight on July 1, 1997.) Similar to the experience I had in Europe just a year and a half back, but Hong Kong presented in a much more metropolitan way, more city, more shiny, more new. Everyone was wearing so much black. Black berets, black blazers, shiny black leather boots, slim black skinny slacks, silky black-patterned blouses and sweaters with stylish scarves, black-rimmed glasses. So much style. This was different from the punk and new wave I had experienced in London. This was classy, sophisticated, and modern.

Soon after Hong Kong, we arrived in Calcutta. My dad stopped at a bookstore in Calcutta's main shopping district Bowbazaar. My family and I entered, and I wandered over to where there were a few western band's cassettes on sale. I bought a cassette to play on my Japanese Walkman. It was The Eurythmics. It was not something I had seen in the US, and it contained some of their older music, including "This Is the House," "The Walk," and "Love Is a Stranger" which would become the soundtrack of the trip.

Soundtracks are important aspects of my life. I utilize music to make different periods, different journeys and physical trips. This period was marked by that first Eurythmics album that I bought bootlegged on the streets of India.

It was around this time I started realizing how big (and interesting) the world was outside the United States, and so far ahead of the US, in so many ways. It is the exact opposite of what we as Americans are raised to believe.

We flew back home after 2 months overseas. I had to hide all the mosquito bites I had been gifted in India. My legs were covered.

A few days after I got back, Hailey and Dolan saw me and came up to me.

"How was it?"

"How was India?"

They were still interested in talking to me. And more importantly, they wanted to hear about my trip. I was excited to share with them the style I had seen in Hong Kong. Surely, they would want to hear about that.

"Oh, it was so cool," I said excitedly. "People are so mod…" I was putting my books away in my locker and began to turn around, but before I could finish, they both rolled their eyes and started laughing.

"Oh god."

They were laughing and shaking their heads as they walked away. Uninterested? Mocking? Perhaps.

"I mean, the style was so cool." I tried to correct myself, but it was too late.

The two of them walked off shaking their heads.

I was left standing there, my words reverberating in my head.

The cool kids, Hailey and Dolan, never spoke to me again.

Plenty
BY MOUSHUMI GHOSE

The abundance of life
The boys and girls who have left
Gaping holes in my heart
Let them be free
Let them fly high
I will
Get on by

Projects will run over
My bucket will spill
My head will be full
Of love and arts
And friends a plenty

❦ Chapter 5 ❧

Come Out, Come Out
Wherever You Are
1987

I was walking towards the bathroom, and there they were on a bench, under the stairs, off to the side. The fluorescent light was shining down bright on them as they made out, lips entwined, legs intertwined. The skinny one with pale skin and long red hair was wearing a red leather jacket and tall black and white striped socks pulled up to her skinny white thighs. The other one had tan skin, dark spiky short hair, white and black socks, and shiny black patent leather shoes. It didn't matter. They were stylish and seductive. Androgynous.

It would be a few months till I would meet them.

It was tricky to get on Eva's radar, initially. She didn't know I was bisexual – I barely knew I was, so I was of no interest to her.

Eva was the dark-haired more masculine presenting one. By then I had a lot of friends at the club and had become quite the regular. I was also meeting up with the kids from other schools on weekdays after school. My friends at the high school who also went to the club were not surprised by my admission, "I think I like Eva."

And yet, some other friends were surprised. That's the thing about coming out. You never know who is and who isn't going to support you. Sometimes people surprise you. You learn a lot about people when you come out.

Queer behavior and lifestyle were still not widely accepted in the 1980's. And there was certainly something about that fact that I liked. I did not want the normative. I knew I needed to rock the boat. This meant something to me, but I didn't know what exactly.

I liked her. Seeing her dance and interacting with all our friends, it awoke something in me. I got caught up in the desire. And my life suddenly felt colorful like I had never seen before. And sound, music seemed so loud. And poetry. So much poetry in my ears. I felt her in a land of darkness, she opened a world to me of vampires and sex appeal. I was aroused by the idea of sexual fluidity and openness. It was all exciting. Euphoric. It all represented freedom.

Then. We would dance. Hundreds of kids from across four counties. We would converge once a week, spilling into the weekend and through Sunday. For dancing. And eyeliner. For hairspray and ecstasy pills. To make out under the strobe lights, in the dark corners. Dance floors and suspenders. Glitter and gold. It was now 1988.

One night I got wind of a house party a lot of the club kids were going to. I invited my adorable friend Miki. She wore all black and lots of chain necklaces. Somehow, even though I assumed Miki was straight, I convinced her to come to the party and pretend that we were girlfriends. Miki, surprisingly, went along with it. People were curious about us, and simultaneously, a few even suspected our game. This was my way of coming out.

Eva was there, sitting quietly with her back to a wall. The other one from under the stairs with long red hair and her red leather jacket was there, too. I learned that her name was

Chloe. And they were surrounded by their cool gang of goth androgynous friends on the couch.

They were so cool.

I wanted to be accepted by them but more so, they awakened in me things which had been dormant. I suddenly knew I was bisexual, but I had no idea how to do go about coming out.

Miki and I walked in holding hands. "This is my girlfriend, Miki." Miki was straight, straight as an arrow, or so I thought. In fact, I thought so for many years despite a lot of contrary evidence, and her eventually coming out to me, many years later.

Introductions ensued.

"This is my girlfriend, Miki," I said again.

Miki had a shy way about her, although she was simultaneously outgoing. She waved as she said, "Hi," and sat down on the floor.

All eyes were on us. More queers, more femme queers. Could this be true? Disbelieving but hopeful.

"You guys are girlfriends?" Chloe shrieked from across the room, with that tone of suspicion.

We both nodded. "Yes," I mumbled, as I sat down next to Miki.

I could feel their eyes on me and their eyes looking at each other exchanging curious glances.

"Let's play a game," Chloe said. She was not going to let this go. She was going in for the kill. "Let's play Truth or Dare."

"Okay."

"Woohoo."

"Yea!"

"I'm in."

More people came and joined our circle.

Chloe was onto me and had tunnel vision on me. "Truth or Dare, Mou!" she screamed from across the room.

True to my scaredy cat nature, and afraid of the sudden interest and spotlight, naturally I chose the safer choice of the two. "Truth."

"Okay," she acquiesced, a tone in her voice saying she wasn't going to let this be easy. "How long have you and Miki been dating?" She was bound to either find holes in our story or shake us to our core until we caved in either direction. Thankfully, Miki and I had already rehearsed this part.

"Six months," I said. And I saw Miki also nodding. "Yep," she mumbled.

We played a few more rounds with the other players who were joining, and then it was back to Chloe. She was not letting us go.

"Truth or dare, Miki."

Miki laughed and said, "Fine, dare."

"Kiss each other," Chloe said.

At this point, Miki laughed nervously and mumbled, "Okay, c'mon." The tone in her voice was more, "Let's get this over with for these incessant children."

We both played on and laughed it off.

But for me the night was filled with tension. Because I wasn't in a relationship with Miki, and I was lying. And we never did kiss.

And now I was going to have to find a way to dig myself out of a lie. If there is anything I suck at, it is lying. All I wanted was to come out. I wanted Eva to know I liked her.

Eventually though, I let it be known. I told some friends who I just knew would spread the word fast. I told them that I had a crush on Eva.

"But, what about Miki?" they asked.

"Oh, we broke up." That was that. The lie was done. Miki and I were done.

It wasn't very long after that when Eva started to pay more attention to me.

A few weeks later, in the parking lot of Denny's, our local hangout, a friend brought me a flower. In this young love, your friends act as go-betweens. This is exciting. This is fun. Sixteen.

"She wants you to have this." My heart was a flurry.

Sixteen. Age of awakening. About love, life and everything in between. So many things new. So many things untouched, untapped, fresh.

"Does she like me?"

"Oh, I think she's totally into you."

I excitedly took the flower and wondered what would come next. We were to meet up.

Her parents were out of town. "She's having a party. She wants you to come over."

A group of us ended up at her house. I wondered how this would go. I had never really hooked up with anyone before. Well, there was that one time a few months before, when I had dry sex on the carpeted bathroom floor, at a party with a boy, a cute boy. I thought he was hot. Later, I kissed another androgynous goth boy, with white hair and eyeliner. That night at her house, I learned that I'm not one to beat around the bush. The longer I waited, the more tedious it felt. So, of course, I finally broke the ice. "What are we doing here?"

We're sitting on the couch. Four of us. Eva and I are sitting between our friends Michael and Joe. I turn to Eva and she and I start making out. She turns me on. Something I have never experienced before. Mike says to Joe, "There's something going on between us." I'm so turned on by Eva. The pun makes us all laugh.

Sex with her. Eyes closed. Clothes on. Hand jobs. Lots of hand jobs. This was perfect for my 16-year-old self. Young love and young sex. As we grow older, we lose that innocence. For example, sex with clothes on. That is hot. I don't care if you're 16 or 60, or what gender you are. Don't lose sight of your innocence. And do try having sex with your clothes on.

The next month carried me along on a cloud. Of love and lust. We wrote each other letters. We wrote each other poetry. I couldn't wait to see her. I was excited and awake. I was in love.

Soon I started noticing small things that felt uncomfortable. For example, the way she bragged about her ex or the way she let people talk down to her.

I found myself getting bored quickly. If she wasn't talking about her ex, or introducing me to obscure music and movies like *The Hunger*, the classic 1980's bisexual vampire movie with David Bowie, and a steamy lesbian sex scene with Susan Sarandon and Catherine Deneuve, then it seemed we had nothing to talk about.

Our relationship lasted for one month. And then we were done. But I was just getting started.

I did the next thing, the break-up part. I got bored, then curious. Chloe had been flirting with me, and I liked her back. I liked her long red hair. Her style. I envisioned us being an attractive femme and adventurous couple.

At Eva's house while Eva was at work, Chloe and I got drunk.

"I'm so sorry," I cried later to Eva, being a huge drama queen.

Eva looked at me with little expression.

"I love you, but I cheated on you with Chloe."

Eva said nothing. In fact, I think she was about to excuse my behavior. Dare I say she might have even liked this?

But I was laying it on thick. I had cheated. That means the end, right?

"I'm so sorry. I do love you, but…"

I did feel bad. I just wanted to have fun and to keep it moving.

Then poof. I was moving on. With the new girl. I had a new girlfriend. Girlfriend number two.

She wore red leather pants and tight leather jackets, with a black fishnet body suit. She wore pointy shoes with buckles. Her hair was long. Dyed. Bright red. She smelled of Poison perfume and hair dye. She drank and swore like a sailor. She was so fucking cool. As cool as can be. Her name was Chloe.

Eva didn't seem too plussed when I told her I'd cheated on her with Chloe. She moved on quickly as well.

Chloe and I were trouble together. We were dangerous and daring, bad influences on each other. I wanted to be like her, sexy and adventurous. I loved her style. I thought she was so cool. I wanted us to be the hot couple. I pictured a different, sexier, cooler, more stylish version of myself.

The first time we fooled around, she cut, dyed and shaved my hair. She would buy me things. This was exciting and new. I could finally have the cool clothes I'd always wanted. I understood then that we could have what we want if we had the means. We would drive into the city and buy all sorts of sexy goth clothes, footwear, lingerie on Haight Street, and at high-end department stores she would pay for them with credit cards, or hard-earned cash given to her by her sugar daddy. Or maybe it was Daddies, plural. I never knew and I never asked. Perfume. Clothes. Anything she wanted. San Francisco was this sexy, wet, gray, dark mystery. Everyone wore black. I was ecstatic. She made and spent a lot of money. I reaped the benefits.

Randomly, she would come to my high school in the middle of the day, driving different fancy cars, and always in the same cool red leather motorcycle outfit. She would bring me lunch, and I would feel so cool, so special.

But things didn't last very long.

I knew that Chloe played in a world I didn't understand, her life and experiences were a little advanced for me. Her world which initially seemed dangerous, mysterious, sexy, and fun, started to feel scary, daunting, and unsafe. Although she was just one year older than me, because she didn't go to school, she had a lot of free time. As a 16-year-old who still lived with my parents, I was only able to join the festivities after school for a few hours and on the weekend. Essentially, I was missing out on a lot of the fun.

Funny how the things we are initially attracted to are the things that will eventually break us apart.

Our mutual friend suddenly started talking about a party they'd had a few nights before.

"You guys had a party?" I asked, feeling the pangs of envy seeping in.

"Yes, on Wednesday night. Miki came over," he said.

"She did?" I was surprised they had a party on a Wednesday night. Not only did I not know about it, but I was also not invited. This wasn't surprising since they probably knew I couldn't come anyway, but it still hurt. Not to mention, they invited my ex-girlfriend, Miki. She was supposed to be my ex! I was floored. I suddenly felt scared, unsure of who I could really trust.

This fun, teenage relationship for a kid who was still in high school was starting to feel outside of my league. I was too young to go out mid-week, stay with friends and have week-long parties like Chloe was doing.

"Yes, we played Truth or Dare. Chloe might have gone down on Miki. Miki also told her you two have never dated."

Might have? You told her what? Not only was I not invited, but I was also mortified and humiliated.

I tried to play it off as though I wasn't hurt, but the truth was I had been uninvited, left out and then cheated on.

The thoughts were swarming. I felt simultaneously betrayed by all three. All in one swoop. It felt like they did this all behind my back. I was so naïve.

I decided to let it go. I had to save face. And, I was determined to have fun. In that moment, I chose to ignore all the ugliness and focus on the fun.

"Well, I'll see you guys on Friday night!" I'd learned my lesson, and I had to let it go.

Friday night was business as usual, and by Sunday things were back to normal. I ignored the betrayals. I knew that come Monday I would be leaving for a month-long trip to the east coast. I was in it for the parties and the parties only.

That Sunday, before I left, I said to Chloe, "Wait for me."

"I will," she said.

She didn't. While I was gone, Chloe moved on.

I came back and we had a final phone call. She was done with me. "We aren't together anymore," she said, spelling it out for me.

"Okay," I said, matter of fact, but I felt my voice quiver. It hurt to hear it. I wished I hadn't called her.

My heart sank to my belly. I was stunned. I held back tears. But, I knew it was for the best.

I knew the relationship had no sustainability before it even started.

Life would have to go on without her.

I gathered myself back up. I wasn't going to let the embarrassment take hold. Now, it was time. I was ready. I was done with this lesbian scene.

And just like that I walked away. My summer of lesbian love ended just as abruptly as it had started.

Chapter 6

Mirror, Mirror on the Floor
1988

I woke up on the couch one early morning late that summer. The sun was rising. I could hear the birds chirping. Except for the sun peering through the trees outside, the rest of the house was still dark from the night.

I must've passed out there on the couch at some point the night before. I was still wearing my clothes from last night. A pair of black shorts. I had on ripped tights underneath, and a black cut-off top that showed off my midriff. Someone must have covered me up with a blanket. How long had I been asleep?

My girlfriend and I and some of our friends had all come over the night before to have a party. But the details of the night were foggy.

Then I remembered. We were planning to party but it was pretty uneventful. My girlfriend encouraged me to rest. "Take a nap," she said.

Right then I heard some laughter and voices. I heard a man's deep voice. Where was everyone?

I walked down the hall of my friend Guy's house and found the room where the voices were coming from. I listened for a moment. I heard Guy's voice and then I heard my friend Kate's voice, mingled with the low voice of a man.

I knocked.

"Come in." It was Guy's voice.

I opened the door to his bedroom to find the 4 of them all sitting around in a circle. The feeling of self-consciousness took over me. Suddenly it felt like all eyes were on me. My friends were there, all three of them from the night before, including my girlfriend and Guy's older brother, Nate.

"Hey Mou," said Kate.

"How'd you sleep?" my girlfriend piped up, laughing.

"Good, I think." Then I asked, "What's going on in here? Why are you guys all up so early?"

My girlfriend and Guy both laughed as I sat down around the circle joining my friends.

"Mou, this is Nate, he lives here."

Nate said hello and as I looked over Nate was making lines of something white on a mirror.

My girlfriend was watching me and said, "Do you want to try some, Mou?"

"Sure."

The next thing I knew Nate who had just put out a line handed me the mirror, and someone handed me a straw. I was still waking up. The warmth of the sleep still around me. The comfort of my friends all around me. I took the plate in my hand and then snorted it.

It was crank. Crank is a form of Meth or Methamphetamine.

***NOTE: I do not recommend you try this – studies show that the side effects of methamphetamine can include addiction and other harmful long-term effects.

A few minutes later, I started to feel great. I was awake, alert and feeling exhilarated.

The four of us talked all morning. I had so much to talk about, so many things to say. All of my so many thoughts and ideas were flowing. I felt excited. I felt alive. I felt exhilarated.

We talked into the afternoon about life, and love and sexuality, and parents and struggles. And truths. So many truths. We listened. We bonded. We connected so deeply for the first time. All of us. We were alive. Really truly alive. We talked all day and then day turned into night. And we kept talking. We talked all weekend.

I lost weight. Now I know this was just water weight. In 24 hours, I lost the extra pounds this chubby girl had always been carrying around for years. Gone. Just like that. I became a skinnier, more self-confident version of myself, literally overnight.

***NOTE: I think it's important to call out skinny culture here. I recognized over the years that many girls would fall prey to a lifestyle involving drugs, specifically uppers and amphetamines like speed, coke, Adderall and the likes which also have the side effect of suppressing appetite and relieving water retention. It's a dirty little secret that too many people know about, unfortunately. The sad part is that these drugs make you feel good, at least initially, and a nice little side effect is it keeps the weight off. For too many people this is a win-win that keeps them stuck in the cycle even when the fun wears off.

That's when the drugs took main stage. My third love in this summer of love. I felt on top of the world, like I finally had a purpose.

I couldn't wait for the weekends. I counted down the days during the week, biding my time at school. On the weekends, we would still meet at the club. Other weekend nights, I would leave my little suburban town to travel to another suburban town, the next county over. Guy's parents were never home so the whole lot of us, a bunch of queer, new wave kids, would pile into his house on weekends.

Back at my high school I found a connection to buying ecstasy from Dave. Dave was this kid with long hair who hung out in the smoking section with all the other heavy metal kids. Suddenly, I was hanging out in the Cancer Cove, the smoking section of the school. (Yes, in the 1980s you could still smoke on campus if you were 16 and older.) I mean, who was I? The 15-year-old and younger me would not recognize this person.

So, the collecting began on Thursday afternoon and evening. I would get the money from my friends. It was $10 a pop, and everyone wanted one. I would sometimes get $150 even $200 from my friends and buy 10-20 hits at 10$ apiece. I would then scrape a little off the top out of each for myself. I justified it as the cost of pick-up and delivery. I went through the trouble to coordinate and get the goods, so the least I could do is get a free hit out of it. So I skimmed the top to get mine. And, we all still had great times.

"Meet me at the parking lot behind the school," Dave said. He lingered before he hung up.

When I drove to meet him, he was already parked, waiting in his Honda Civic. Dave was cute in the All-American boy, rock 'n' roll Tom Petty kind of way. Not my style really, as these days I preferred the eye-lined types. Dave had longish hair on the sides. He wore ripped jeans, a white, Pink Floyd T-shirt. I got out of my car. It was 6 PM on a Friday evening, I was going straight to Kate's house to pick her up and meet up with the rest for a fun weekend. I was already dressed for the club. I had on black short shorts, black tights, pointy shoes, a gray vest and the reddest lipstick I could find.

I got out of my car to meet him, and he got out to greet me. At school he was always aloof and short, but today he smiled at me. He must have liked what he saw. And, as we exchanged the drugs and the money, I gestured the money towards him as he reached out to slide the drugs into my hand and do the trade. Our hands touched one another briefly and then there it was, he smiled at me again, twice in one day, giving me that knowing glance. It was official. I had a crush on my drug dealer.

But I was off and running. I had no time to waste on this waif-like pale rock 'n' roll boy at my high school. I was on my way to see my pretty boys and pretty girls, all decked out in their 1980's new wave make-up and goth clothing of fishnets and hairspray, ties and boots. Where fashion met music, and everyone was waiting for me to bring the drugs and to bring the fun!

I hightailed it out of there and I realized in that moment how my life had changed so fast. I had suddenly, overnight it seemed, outgrown high school.

Ecstasy and speed were bonding drugs. We came alive. We were oh so glamorous. And, we were having the time of our life.

And as the weeks sped up and I lived for the weekends, I barely noticed that my girlfriend and I had broken up. I had more important things to do, like drugs and hanging out with my new friends. We would experiment with LSD, mushrooms, and cocaine. I had a huge group of friends who accepted me for who I was. All the harsh criticism and judgment of my past fell away for the first time and led me to this place where everyone and everything was accepted. This was the queer community, and the drugs amplified that effect. Everyone could finally show up as themselves. It was exhilarating.

And everything was suddenly okay.

Wild and Queer Girls
BY MOUSHUMI GHOSE

We tossed boys out our windows
while the gals came flying in
throngs
hordes
with their whiskey and Obsession
tall tales and long legs
of
late nights and compersion

No time to waste
on hatred or envy
on straight poop misery
or hetero-normativity
boring, Sydney, boring
The boys, they wanted to own us.
We said, Nope.
Be us.
Nope.
Join us.
Well, okay, maybe.
For a minute or two
As long as you behave yourself, act cool
check your toxicity of the masculine sort at the door
or get checked
then get the boot
If you fail to follow suit
or argue back like an idiot
proving us right

We fought for so long
against the man
the literal man
holding each other up
wild and queer girls
Bisexual, Pan and Lesbian
Sisters looking out for each other
Baby dykes, butch and femmes
Sisters one for all
All till Fall
for one day will be gone.

∞ Chapter 7 ∞

Fair-Weathered Friends
or Different Values
1988

I was having a lot of fun. I was now starting to call myself bi. I was so excited to finally have a friend group that prioritized fashion, style, and music. Something I had been missing my entire 16 years of life. For the first time, I felt like I was living the life I was meant to be living.

My newfound friends were on the wild side. On the outside, everyone dressed in either all black, with dyed black hair or were inspired by some other new wave fashion choices. It was common to dye or have bleached hair, also common were shaved sides, shaved underneath, lots of hairspray and the new wave styles including leather biker jackets, chokers around the neck, studded bracelets, fishnet stockings, and pleather, lots of pleather. The styles were not what you could simply buy off a rack from a department store, not unless you had a lot of money and you were shopping in the city. Out here in the suburbs, it required a certain amount of savvy and a whole lot of creativity to put together these styles. This is what I was drawn to. I was ready to embrace this in my life fully.

It had been a few years already that I had been sewing my own clothes, to be able to create styles that weren't found in our local JC Penny's or Sears stores. I would get mom to take me to the fabric store and I would buy fabric to make myself long pencil skirts. I got some cute black buckled boots from Express, and I would wear my dad's oversized sweaters. That was in the eighth grade. Now I was in the tenth grade, and I no longer had the time, nor the interest to make my own clothes anymore. As my social life became more demanding, much to my mom's chagrin, I started shopping at thrift stores.

This crowd of people understood my sense of style, even though I was having a hard time pulling it off. Most of the time my hair would not cooperate, and frankly I was just a bit chubby to achieve the way I wanted it to. Still, this gave me something to aspire to.

Sian, my friend at school, was not happy with this. Neither was my mom.

Aside from shopping at thrift stores, my mom would ask, "Why would you want to wear something that someone else wore before when we can afford new clothes?" My mom thought these friends were bad news. She'd say, "Always hanging around. Where are their parents? When do they study?" My mother was very concerned that I was falling in with the wrong crowd. And she was right. I was *finally* falling in with the wrong crowd! But they were the right crowd for me.

Sian was clearly threatened. "Who are your real friends?" Sian asked me. Wow! Straight to the point. I felt like I had been punched in the gut.

I wondered if she was right. But simultaneously I felt unsupported and unseen. I thought Sian knew me, knew what I stood for. That this wasn't just some phase of trying to fit in, this was who I was destined to be.

Was I truly making bad choices and hanging out with people who weren't my true friends? I couldn't help feeling that maybe she was right. I think somewhere I knew these weren't the most ambitious of friends, at least academically speaking, but that's not to say they weren't trying to achieve things. Fashion and music were perhaps more important. And having fun. Meeting people. Going out. We were just different. And, the truth was I was losing interest in our friendship, and so I was exchanging her for a crowd of people. But, were they my true friends? I was doubting myself.

And to top it off, when Sian was around, my mother, who was also having a hard time understanding all my (bad) choices, which were seemingly getting worse, would throw me under the bus. "Sian, who are these friends of Mou's?" Which only gave Sian more fuel when it came to the assassination of my character and my newfound friends group. My mom was at her wit's end trying to keep me straight in line. And, while my mom was acting completely inappropriately, and having poor boundaries by asking my peer this question about my other peers, I gave my mother a pass. She is my mother after all. Calling her out about outing me to Sian was not a fight worth having.

But Sian was a different story altogether. She was not my mother. She was not even my family. She was my peer. And she was my peer from school. She could not pass go and collect $200, not that easily.

What sucked for me, is I had expected more from her. I mistakenly thought her to be more like me. I thought we had more in common. I thought she would understand.

Sian and I had become friends at the end of my freshman year. I spotted her in an assembly. She had on glasses that were decorated with stickers. She had long hair. In that moment I thought to myself, stickers on her glasses? Okay, dork.

But, lo and behold, Sian pursued a friendship with me. She was athletic and hung out with the academic types. She was on the debate team and the drama club. She was one of those kids who was good at everything. And, as someone who didn't quite fit in with any of those groups, I didn't feel like I had anything in common with her. I was not athletic nor academic, I didn't debate nor act. I hung out with the new wave kids, the smokers with the punk rock hair. We listened to what the kids today call goth music. Sian and I were so different.

One day while she was befriending me, she discovered some lyrics handwritten by me on the paper bag book cover of my text book.

"Cool," she said.

That was when I finally started to let my guard down. A girl in my otherwise homogeneous and suburban high school who also liked song lyrics. What were the chances? Maybe we did have something in common after all. Maybe we could be friends.

Plus, Sian was persistent. Okay, why not give her a chance? I needed more friends anyway. I wasn't going to turn down friends.

Sian and I started doing a lot together. We were into Astrology, and I was able to share my love of music and poetry with her, to some degree. Though she was only surface interested, I introduced her to bands like The Smiths and R.E.M.

Being one of the top athletes at the school in girls' soccer and volleyball, she was in good shape, while I, a slacker artist type, was kind of chubby with bad hair. She knew I felt that way, down about my appearance and she would often play up her attractiveness, which should have tipped me off to the kind of person she was. Honestly, in my self-degradation, I was kind of hoping to hear different words such as, "You're not chubby," or, "You're pretty with good style," yea, so maybe I was fishing. But she never uttered those words, which only validated my teenage insecurities, and in hindsight should have been a red flag.

Still, we were close. We rode bikes to each other's houses and spent the long days of summer going back and forth to each other's house. Sure, Sian and I had a lot of fun, but admittedly I wanted more. I wanted intrigue, excitement, music, and color in my life. I wasn't an athlete, and I didn't hang out with the brainy kids so much. I was a bad girl in my heart. I wanted to smoke cigarettes and wear black eyeliner, look cool, intimidate people and write goth music. Sian wasn't interested in any of that. And, the one thing that I was good at, which was piano, was something that Sian was also good at. Go figure. She made sure when I played piano, she would one up me on how good she was.

But I was an aspiring writer, and I read her my dark poetry, inspired by the music I was listening to. I was hoping for some kind words, like the day we first met, something to validate my art and in turn, me. Instead, I got, "I am worried about you." It was starting to feel like I was there to build Sian up. She was there to tear me down.

Sian was interested in boys though, and was crushing on one boy, so we would bond over that. I was interested in boys, especially if they were cute boys. But, ultimately while Sian was funny and nice, I didn't feel like we had a lot in common. This became more and more obvious as I drifted further and further away into what was considered the world of darkness.

One day, several months later, I decided to break the news to her. We had drifted quite far apart and I was tired of her passive aggressive comments about my friends. But that summer right before senior year, I had become involved with females, and was having the best summer of my life. I was exploring my sexuality and really wanted to share it with her, my good friend Sian, the way we used to talk about wanting boyfriends. I had had sexual experiences with women and had girlfriends.

"I've discovered that I am bisexual," I said eagerly, awaiting her response. Followed by, "I fell in love with a woman this summer." I foolishly expected her to be supportive. Hadn't we shared so much, our crushes, our desires? She would be happy for me, right?

Instead, she said, with nary a smile on her face, "You really should not be flaunting that." I was aware enough to know, this was her anger talking. I knew Sian wasn't homophobic, she was hurt. But I was thrown for a loop. This language felt toxic and demeaning.

I didn't have words for it back then, but I knew this was not someone I could be friends with any longer. She had withdrawn all support, and what had once been subtle insults became putting me down to my face. If this was her way of staying friends, it was backfiring terribly! Not to mention the even bigger issue of homophobia. Here I was hanging out with a decidedly queer group, and that she could say something so cruel, unkind and homophobic kind of blew me away. This was it – a moment of truth. As a feminist, homophobia had no place in women's liberation.

This moment drove the nail home. At that moment, I knew what I had known all along. We had nothing in common from day one. Heartbroken and sad, I never shared anything else with Sian.

In the months that followed, she proceeded to try to hurt me in other ways. Dare I say she was obsessed with it?

We had become Teen Advocates, a program we had applied to prior to me meeting my lovers and dabbling in drugs. Teen Advocates would speak to Junior High Kids about the dangers of drugs. We even had to sign something that said we would not do drugs. I took an oath. Yet here I was using drugs on the weekends. Speed, ecstasy, cocaine, rush. Sian didn't know for sure, but she knew the crowd I was hanging with, and she could certainly make an educated guess. But, instead of talking to me about it, she decided to attempt to out me to my class by asking an anonymous question at our Teen Advocates meeting.

The decorated box was passed around and everyone was to drop a question, a comment, something nice to say to someone into the box when it came around. Then we all went around and pulled something out of the box and read it aloud.

Suddenly someone was reading out loud from a piece of paper, directly to me: "Mou," my ears perked up, and even before the words came out of the student's mouth, I knew in my heart what was coming next…

"Is it true that you do drugs on the weekends?" There it was. I was on the spot. I felt the blood drain from my face, and my palms went cold. I acted confused, shocked, and surprised. Everyone's eyes were on me. And, the worst part, I just knew it was Sian who put this question into the box.

Embarrassed and simultaneously angry at Sian's pettiness, I responded, "Oh my gosh, what the? No way!" I lied. "I have never ever tried drugs in my life." Although yes, I had begun using ecstasy, and even buying it for all my friends at the underground club. I knew I was being a hypocrite. But, Sian could have talked to me about anything and all of it nicely at any given point. We might have had a different outcome.

I left the meeting that day and never talked to Sian after that. My head was reeling. I was worried I would get caught. I couldn't believe she would stoop so low. No, I could. I had known from day one, but I had decided to doubt my own intuition. That was it. I was always doubting my own intuition.

Eventually, I quit the Teen Advocates, citing that I was 'just too busy.'

Yes, I was too busy. Too busy for the rigid rules of the day. Yes, I was doing drugs. I was also exploring my sexuality. I was busy making friends who accepted me, flirting, running amok with shenanigans, some innocent and some not so much, getting into all kinds of trouble and simultaneously learning so much. Lots of life lessons about young love, friendships, sexuality, and more. As a teen still living at home I could see how one might think I was acting out dangerously, in which case Sian wasn't wrong about outing me, but the fact that she knew I was finally living in a way that felt authentic and priceless to me, and then still wanting to rain on that parade told me everything I needed to know about her.

True friends want the best for each other, even if it hurts. That's what I have always believed.

I want to add that one size does not fit all when it comes to substance use. The old adage "Say No To Drugs" is fine, and understandably important to those who have problems with controlling their drug use. But this one size fits all idea of abstinence is also damaging. I acknowledge that drug misuse and abuse exist. I have many friends and loved ones who have been affected in terrible ways. I also know many folks who practice mindfulness and use of substances in mindful and deliberate ways, which are not abusive nor maladaptive. This should not be shamed. As we know, shaming is harmful. Often drug use is borne out of chronic trauma that exists in one's environment. Healing is also not always linear and cut-and-dry. There is a term for this mindful use of substances. It's called 'harm-reduction.' The harm reduction model is rooted in social justice and creates space for dialogue and movement towards fluidity, healing the harms caused by racialized drug policies which can sometimes do more harm than good.

❦ Chapter 8 ❧

The Truth Behind the Candy
1989

It was something to do. Senior year in high school was turning out to be a little less fun and sexually explorative than last year had been. So, no harm, right?

I got ready. It was always hard getting ready in the hot suburb. The weather in San Francisco was always much colder. Still, I was looking forward to a night out with Regina and some of her friends.

Regina had this friend Lola. I had actually met Lola when we were younger about 3 or 4 years back when I was in junior high school. (In junior high and high school 4 years feels like a lifetime.) Lola and I had walked around the music festival together. Eating cotton candy, talking about new wave music and fashion. We bonded. She seemed like she was a cool, music loving girl like me. A feminist. A girl's girl. We're not necessarily lesbians, but we put the sisterhood, friendship and other women first. We certainly don't put men ahead of us. But in the 1980's, things were more binary. Girls either liked boys and were boy crazy or they were the opposite: man hating lesbians. The irony is that before adolescence we were allowed to exist on a spectrum, outside binary. And that's where we were that day at the fair.

I was excited to get reconnected to Lola. We were in high school now, and I was excited to find out that she and Regina were close friends. *What a small world!*

Regina and I had met just last year when she dated a mutual friend, at the tail end of my relationship with Chloe.

But after Chloe and I split up, I no longer had that clout. Besides, most of my female friends identified as straight, so now I was just a weird lesbian in their eyes.

I had called Regina the afternoon that Chloe had ended it and said, "Guess what?"

"What?" Regina asked.

"I'm free," I said.

She was quiet. "What do you mean?"

"Chloe and I broke up. I'm free."

"Oh, are you okay?" Regina was trying to sound caring, but underneath it she sounded non-plussed.

"Yea, for sure. I feel great." I was looking for reassurance. I needed to hear, "You don't need her." Or even just, "Good for you." I was looking for a friend. But there was very little said. My heart sank at that moment. I imagined I sounded like I was trying to cover up my sadness. Maybe I was. I was looking for camaraderie, and what I ended up feeling in the moment was alone. The thing that had brought so much excitement into my life, and set me apart even, was gone. I was alone and unimportant. Uncool.

"What else is going on?" Regina asked. And, that was it. I was no longer Mou and Chloe.

Still, I was hopeful.

"Let's hang out."

After that, I started spending even more time with Regina. Regina and I had fun. We both enjoyed going to parties, and we had all the gay boys in common. She even tolerated the lesbians.

"What's going on tonight?"

"Lola and I are going to Club Metro. Do you want to come with us?"

I met Regina and Lola at Lola's place. Immediately I could sense the vibe was tense, hectic. It didn't feel warm and welcoming.

"Lola, this is Mou, you remember her?"

"Oh hey, yea, how are you?" Lola kept a straight face, looked me up and down then proceeded to do her make-up.

I wanted to respond, *I'm good, it's been forever, and how cool is it that we both know Regina,* but before I had the chance, I realized Lola had no intention of engaging in conversation with me as she continued to address Regina.

"He has so much money, but he knows better than to fuck with me. He knows what's good for him." Lola put her brightest red lipstick on and admired herself in the mirror as she spoke. She continued, "I think you'll really like him."

Regina's eyes lit up. "Cool." She got up to pour herself a drink. "Let's go have some fun." Lola barely even acknowledged my existence.

Both Regina and Lola were wearing slinky dresses and high-heeled shoes. I felt out of place in my new wave club outfit and big clunky club shoes.

Lola came back out into the living room and handed me a straw. "Do you want some?"

"Sure!" I never said no to party favors and I was eager to bond with Lola and Regina.

One thing I knew though was that nose candy was the great leveler. It made everyone bond. It made everyone look beautiful and alive. At least temporarily. And I needed that.

We were off to the races. And my club outfit suddenly looked and felt a lot sexier.

Lola drove us to San Francisco in her parent's car. Things were feeling much better now that we were high. I felt more confident and joined the conversation more readily. I was comfortable, able to enjoy myself, though I did notice the conversation did tend to center around men, finding the rich ones, and who was who at the club. Lola clearly knew some people and wanted to introduce Regina to some men. I guessed I was the wing woman. Despite the confidence from the drug, I had the intuition and feeling of not being in the right place.

As the night wore on, it was clear that Lola was no longer that warm and friendly, feminist girl I'd met at the music festival. Back then she was interested in music and I got the impression she was like me, eager to dismantle the patriarchy. But today she was the complete opposite with her conversation about rich men, her sexy clothes meant to appease the male gaze and her complete disregard for me. She dated older guys and was proud of herself for giving them a run for their money. If I hadn't been trying so hard to be accepted that night, to find my footing after my breakup with Chloe, which was proving to be more demoralizing than I had realized, and to make some female friends I may not have hung around. But instead I remained hopeful.

I wasn't sure why Regina had invited me. Lola seemed pretty preoccupied with herself. I figured that was why. Then I realized Regina was the sidekick, wing woman, and me, I guess I was the ugly duckling tag-along friend.

We got to the club and stood in line. It was 21 and over. Lola wasn't having it and went to the doorman to find her friends, to capitalize on her connections. Before I knew what was going on, we were ushered to the front of the line.

"Come on," Lola motioned to Regina. Of course, I followed.

They were about to let Regina and Lola in and I was there, too. Like a sitting duck. Regina had invited me, but Lola had not.

The doorman asked for my ID.

"ID?"

I didn't have one, and I got turned away from the door.

"Sorry, we can't let you in without a valid ID." Regina and Lola were already inside. Regina looked back at me, shrugged and said, "Sorry."

She invited me, and possibly never even inquired if I could also get in. "Go to Lola's," she yelled, and then she walked into the club and disappeared. I know she was trying to be helpful, but it wasn't enough. It was the sign of someone who is not a true friend.

I stood there stunned. Did Regina and Lola really just go into the club and leave me outside by myself? I felt the eyes on me, as glamorous club goers standing in line watched me get rejected by the door guy, and also my friends.

It was late by now, almost 11 PM. I was in the city, 30 miles away from home. The drugs had worn off and I was just the underage, plain, frumpy, goth girl from the burbs. The truth about the nose candy was staring me in the face. It was all fake. Drugs were a lie.

Embarrassed, I slowly turned around, trying to act as nonchalant as possible and started walking, as if I'd had somewhere else to go. Truth of the matter is I never even asked where we were going. I just went along for the ride. Driven by boredom and a need for excitement is never a good idea. The train ran until 1 AM and I had taken it many times to and from the city. I just had to walk towards Market Street to find a station.

As I walked the shame and humiliation slowly started to melt away. As did the fear of walking after dark in the city. I was suddenly overcome by a sense of overwhelming calm and freedom. The city was electric. There were people everywhere. I didn't want to be in that club with those girls, trying to hook up with rich older men. I was barely 18. I had come out as bisexual. I was not wearing a slinky dress and high heels. I didn't want what toxic masculinity and femininity preyed on. And, in that moment I knew I was going to be okay.

I just had to find my tribe. I knew people like me were out there. On those cool, dark, city streets, I could feel it. And, in that moment I also knew who I didn't want to be friends with. Women like Lola and Regina. Women who were out for themselves and did not have other women's backs.

❧ Chapter 9 ❧

Wake-Up Call
1989

I met Elizha while I was dating my first girlfriend Eva. Elizha was blonde, stylish, and thin. Eliza was the kind of girl who I would want to be friends with but in my past life wouldn't have given me the time of day.

One of my newfound friends was John. He was gay and wealthy. He came from an affluent and educated family from Marin County, and today he had invited us all over to his place for the weekend. His parents were out of town.

John would make his way out to where we lived in the East Bay most weeks. He was one of the first guys in the group who made me feel welcome. He was funny and loud and we immediately hit it off. John was always around. It was hard to conceive that he lived so far away. But, I got the impression that his family were typical for wealthy families; too busy to know what their kids were up to.

So it was a treat to finally get to see where John lived. We knew he lived far away, but we were never privy to what his life really looked like.

I arrived at the party with some of my local friends who had known John from before. For them this was a reunion as they already knew other people at the party. I did not really know anyone besides John and the people I arrived with.

I moseyed my way around the lavish house. It was clear that John's family had a lot of money. I also realized how little I knew about Johns' life. I got the feeling John was often running away from his life. As I looked around the party, I got the sense that most of these people were a little more conservative than our anything goes crowd. I began to understand that John cherished his friends and needed the gay community that we were all a part of, as it was lacking over here in his neck of the woods.

I wandered out onto the back porch, holding my drink, and I was immediately approached by a waify looking girl wearing a blue and white striped shirt and a scarf around her neck. She looked as though she should have been holding a baguette and wearing a beret.

"Hi! I'm Elizha! What's your name?"

Startled a bit at her friendliness, and trying to match her level of enthusiasm I said, "Hi, I'm Mou," and shot her a somewhat forced smile.

"Nice to meet you, Mou!" She gave me a big hug "Where are you from?"

"Oh I came with Kate. I live in Walnut Creek."

"Oh nice! Yea, John always goes, and I have been wanting to join him forever. I have heard a lot about you."

I was feeling flattered that she had taken such an interest in me.

"So tell me more about yourself. Are you dating anyone? What are you into?"

We sat down and talked, and of course, I told her about Eva. It was the early days of dating Eva and I was head over heels, feeling full of joy and so much love for Eva. Eva and I used to write each other little letters and love notes, and she had stolen my heart. I was in love and was able to share that with Elizha so openly. It was nice to be able to tell a female friend all about her.

"Oh that's so wonderful!"

The night ended pretty early as we all had to drive back to the east bay and as I was leaving Elizha came and found me.

"So nice to meet you, Mou." She squeezed me as she hugged me. She smelled like apricots. "Take care of your girl Eva!"

She was all smiles.

"So nice to meet you, Elizha. Come down so we can hang out sometime."

I was glowing. I had met a beautiful young girl who had shown interest in me and showed me so much support for my same sex relationship, as well as the love I was feeling. I felt I had truly met a good friend.

A whole year would pass until I would see Elizha again. In my head and in my heart I always thought of Elizha as a good friend and couldn't wait to reconnect with her in the future.

By senior year, I had broken up with Eva and I was single again. I was single and sowing my oats, hanging out with all sorts of people, and hooking up with boys and girls.

One weekend towards the very end of summer, John invited a bunch of us up to his family's beach house. We drove out in the late night, through dark windy roads out to the sea. We were listening to Depeche Mode's Violator album which had just come out last year.

We finally got to the beach house after 1 AM. John and some of his buddies were gone by the time we got there. In his place was his school buddy, Felix. Felix was heterosexual and attractive. He had tanned skin and was wearing white shorts and a white T-shirt. Although he had a decidedly athletic look about him, which was not my type, he still made a blip on my radar, so he must've been quite good looking.

He immediately began flirting with me, and I him. For the record, I am not a very good flirt. I am down to earth and very matter-of-factly in my demeanor. I guess when I am drunk or high I may act differently, but my usual self is a little less animated.

That night I was really into Felix. We were hanging out with each other all night. Of course, I was high, and I was enjoying just being playful with him, but I wasn't interested, nor was I ready for that matter to have intercourse with him. Finally, we lay down together in the bed. The bed was in a cubby since we were basically in a boat house. We had all our clothes on and the making out and fingering ensued.

I must've fallen asleep because the next thing I knew, I woke up and it was morning. Felix was not in the bed next to me. The lake house was quiet. From where I sat I saw Guy passed out on the couch and some other friends were curled up on the twin beds in the next room. I got up, walked around and wandered into the master bedroom. That was when I saw Felix and Kate lying in bed together.

It was like a scene from a bad movie where the wife or the husband walks in and sees their partner in bed with someone else. Except I barely knew Felix.

Kate and Felix looked up as I walked in and looked terribly guilty. I took one look and my reaction was just as cliché as you see in those movies. I had to catch my breath. I was stunned. Holding back my utter humiliation, I turned around to walk out. I heard Kate say, "Mou, wait…" And then I heard her saying something else, "It's not like you guys were gonna…" and then her voice trailed off.

I wasn't exactly upset or angry, more than anything I was embarrassed. Because I thought Felix liked me when he probably was just looking to get laid. Oh well, I thought, time to go.

I went back to where my stuff was, and I started putting on my shoes. Kate and Felix both followed me out there, and Felix sat down behind me and watched me while I put my shoes on. He may have tried to touch my hair, but I was too embarrassed to engage.

"It's cool," I said.

Then I grabbed my stuff and turned to Guy and said, "Let's go!"

I was ready to let it go, just as much as they were. I did not know Felix before last night, and while we had a wonderful night of connecting, it wasn't like we were going to be boyfriend and girlfriend. I was ready to move on. I knew that I would forgive Kate of this, as we'd been friends for a long time. And, that I would probably never see Felix ever again.

After that incident, no one ever brought it up again. Except Elizha. I decided to call her one afternoon. I had never seen Elizha in person since the first time we'd met, but we talked on the phone from time to time, always trying to find a time to reconnect in person. We always said we would.

Elizha answered the phone.

"Hello?"

"Hey, Elizha, it's Mou." There was a long silence. This was not the warm hello I was expecting.

"Ugh. Why are you calling me?" Her voice was cold.

"Oh, just to say hi!" I tried to sound chipper although I was keenly aware she did not sound happy to hear from me.

"Ugh. I heard what happened with Felix." Then she said, "I thought you were a lesbian."

"Well, I'm bisexual. I like boys and girls."

"Well, I don't get it." She sounded angry. "I have to go."

And just like that, she hung up.

My head was spinning, and I suddenly felt like I had to vomit. Was Elizha upset I had hooked up with Felix? Or, was she upset that I wasn't the lesbian girl, who was in love with Eva, like she thought I was?

Coming out as queer in a mostly heterosexual world is profoundly traumatizing. As I have already mentioned you get support from places you'd never guess and rejected by people who you thought for sure would support you. You really learn the truth about people and who they are by their reactions, which can sometimes be extremely devastating.

You also learn a thing or two about our culture, and in this case:

1) The binary rules that we operate within. Perhaps it was assumed because of my gayness, that I wouldn't care if Kate and Felix hooked up. I was a lesbian after all.

and

2) Toxic competition that can exist between women, fighting for men.

Never in a million years did I think I would get rejected for heterosexual behavior.

೫ Chapter 10 ೪

Mary Ward Hall
1990

I would often joke that I was raised in Mary Ward Hall.
I arrived on a Sunday in the early fall. The next day was to
be the first day of school. My first day at university. And,
my first time ever living away from home.

Naturally, I was scared. Despite having attended the
orientation a few weeks earlier, which I had gone to and
driven to by myself, and although I had been going to San
Francisco regularly for social events with my friends, I let my
parents drive me to the campus housing. My little sister came
too.

I didn't have much with me. I had a couple of suitcases
full of clothes. I didn't know what else to bring. I didn't know
what to expect.

I did not bring my car with me. My expectation of life
was that I would be spending most of my time on campus,
right? Plus living in San Francisco meant I would walk
everywhere, take the bus or public transportation because
parking and driving would be ridiculously hard.

There were three on-campus housing buildings, plus
another fancier apartment building for graduate students. My
building was called Mary Ward Hall.

As could be expected in a big city university, which was also known to be a commuter school, parking was difficult. We had to drive around the campus looking for parking for a good 25 minutes. When we finally parked, we had to walk to get to the building where I would be living. My family and I walked in carrying all of my belongings. Lots of students were milling around the on-campus housing area, socializing, talking with one another. To me, it seemed obvious that I was the new kid on the block with all my belongings and entire family in tow.

We found my room on the 6th floor and introduced ourselves to my new roommate. Her name was Melissa. She was Japanese-American, and her black T-shirt read, "I only wear black." She was welcoming and kind.

My mother began making my bed and giving me suggestions to organize my side of the room. My dad chit chatted with Melissa, while my sister just stood around watching. About an hour later, after unloading everything, and seeing that I had a new roommate I needed to get to know, my parents finally left, and left me to settle in.

I sat down on the bed. What was I to do next?

In one swift move I had gone from being a cool 18-year-old suburban party girl who drove herself all around the bay area for all manner of social affairs, to living in a small dorm room that I shared with a complete stranger. My mother had adorned my twin sized dorm bed with old unattractive bedding from the 1970's she had sitting around. I had never lived away from home, so I allowed her to do so. But, alas I was a big girl in a big city.

Melissa and I talked for a little bit. She had a cynical way of talking and was a bit unsure of herself. We shared some common interests in music.

We spent the evening together. Per my suggestion, we took a walk to get to know the lay of the land. Once outside her social awkwardness hit me. She was an introvert.

We walked up to campus. I checked out where my classes would be the next day and we walked back to our dorm room as it got dark. I checked out the washroom and learned that our floor, the 6th floor, was an all-girls floor.

I sat down in the window, bored, wondering how I was going to make friends, while having a mind-numbing boring conversation with Melissa. Then I looked down and in the dorm room below me, there was an elbow sticking out. It was a male arm.

I turned to Melissa and whispered as I pointed, "Look."

Melissa came over to the window and looked down. She pulled herself back in the room and looked at me quizzically. "That's someone's arm. So?"

"So, let's send them a note!" I said.

She looked perplexed but intrigued. "Okay." Then she said, "We could use a hanger or…" Turns out solving mysteries was where Melissa shined. Then she pulled out a long piece of yarn she happened to have stashed in her crafting kit.

We wrote a note saying, "Hi, we are your upstairs neighbors Mou and Melissa," attached it to the string and then Melissa sent it down. I was too chicken. So, I had Melissa do the dirty work.

A few minutes later, someone tugged on the string and a new note was attached. Melissa pulled the string back up and retrieved the new note.

"Hi, we are Graham and Josh, come over."

Melissa and I looked at one another and giggled like schoolgirls. "Should we?" We both looked at each other. "Why not? What have we got to lose?!"

I realized we were being invited to go meet some boys.

And I sure felt awkward going with Melissa on a blind double date.

But when we got downstairs, I was relieved to see there were already two other non-white females, sitting in the room. I was so relieved. This was no double date at all.

"Hi, I'm Mou."

"I'm Melissa."

There was Graham, Josh and the two gals were Margaret and Lucia.

"I'm Margaret." She held out her hand and smiled.

"Hi! I'm Lucia." Followed by, "Do I know you? I feel like I know you. You look so familiar."

"You look familiar to me, too."

As it turned out Lucia and I did not know each other, per se, but we both may have attended an underage club at the same time. No surprise there, as we were all from the Bay Area. In that moment, I understood what it meant to be at a commuter school.

Lucia and I immediately bonded as kindred spirits. Sometimes you just speak the same language as someone and it clicks. And, as we all hung around there in Josh's and Graham's small dorm room, I suddenly knew everything was going to be okay.

Just a few days after I met Lucia and Margaret, I began meeting more and more people at Mary Ward Hall.

Life in the dorms was wholesome, sweet, and, we definitely partied a lot, too. There were late night study groups in the lounge with chocolate chip cookies and coca cola. Turns out life in the dorms was fun.

It seemed that moving to SF to attend college was the best thing I ever did to get away from the homogenous bubble of suburbia. The dorms were full of all kinds of people, of so many colors and cultures. It was such a melting pot. I had been missing this my entire life.

People complimented my looks. This was new. I had never really experienced this in my 18 years. Had I grown into my looks? Had I finally arrived in a place that appreciated my skin color? Was it because I was in a place of higher education? Perhaps I finally found people who were finally able to openly compliment one another without it being a negative thing. Regardless, it was a definite self-esteem booster. People asked about my culture, with genuine curiosity. In fact, for the first time in my life, I would run into people who actually knew something, anything, about my culture, my background, just by looking at me.

"You're Indian, right?"

"Yes!"

"Which part of India are you from?"

"My parents are from Calcutta."

"Oh, so are you Bengali?"

That people knew anything about India when they weren't Indian was a profound shift, a thing I'd never experienced.

This was a world where diversity was seen as a positive thing.

I was surprised, pleasantly. Culture shock. I decided to lean in. I could finally lean in. Relax. Breathe.

In San Francisco, I was home.

⮞ Chapter 11 ⮜

Straight Poop
1990-1991

Meeting Sally was like a breath of fresh air.

I had only been in the dorms a few weeks and was making my rounds. Getting to know people. I was in San Francisco, but I felt like I was miles away from anyone, any world, any life, I had ever known. I guess I wanted it that way, and it was exciting.

Since my short stint dating girls in high school, I had kind of gone back into the closet. I still had a lot of gay male friends but did not have a single bi or gay female friend to speak of. Once I'd broken up with the girls, I was back to square one. Alone.

Being queer in the early 1990's was not easy. It was downright isolating. And without the support of my queer community, my feminism was falling flat on its face. The straight world was busy perpetuating all sorts of binary and unspoken rigid rules steeped in toxic masculinity and femininity, and I was struggling for air.

I loved Sally's style. She had curly blonde hair and a distinct Madonna vibe about her. (I am talking early 1980's version Madonna.)

Her roommate was Harriet. Harriet was a lesbian and was out. She was a tall blonde Latinx woman who, turns out, knew some of the old crew from the underground club. My world was getting smaller.

Those early days in the dorms at San Francisco State when we would meet someone for the first time, the conversation would often go something like this:

"Hey, I'm {insert name here}, is this your first year?"

"Yep."

"Right on. Where did you live before this?"

"I'm from Walnut Creek."

"Oh cool, I'm from Santa Rosa."

All of this, I suppose, should be prefaced with a disclaimer about life on campus. People live on campus for the sole purposes of: 1) Convenience and 2) The "College Experience" which translates to "I want to meet people." Everyone in the dorms was readily available to meet you. It was easy to make new friends in the dorms. That was why we were all there.

SFSU was a commuter school, as was told to me, and a large majority of the students hailed from somewhere around the Bay Area, and of course you had your smatterings of students from Los Angeles, Southern California, Oregon, New York and other countries.

Harriet was the first person I met who would make my world start to seem small.

When we met in those first few weeks at the dorms, she looked at me inquisitively as we shook hands.

"You look really familiar. Do you know someone by the name of Pierre James?"

"Oh my god, yes!! I love Pierre so much! How do you know him?"

"We met him a few times, but I think we saw you at the Depeche Mode concert, and you were there with him?"

"Oh my god, totally! How cool that you know some of those friends."

Suddenly I had kindred spirits at SFSU. I suddenly felt a glimpse of what my life could be like.

A few days later, I would bump into Harriet down in the cafeteria. She was quiet. Her eyes were intense, and she spoke to you in a very deliberate way.

"Mou, are you gay?"

"Well, I identify as bi, I guess. I dated a couple girls in high school."

"Sally is bisexual too."

"She is?" I didn't believe it. Weren't gay people always trying to say that everyone was gay? I know I would be super excited if that were the truth, but I was finding it difficult to believe Harriet's words.

"Yes, she is. She has a girlfriend. Ask her." Harriet sat down and began eating her food. She was done having this conversation with me.

My mind was still questioning. There was no way that Sally was bisexual. She was way so stylish and feminine. My stereotyping judgment was showing. I still didn't believe lesbians could be stylish and cool, even though I had already dated a couple of them.

The next time I saw Sally, it was business as usual. We made small talk.

"Hey, Sally."

"Hey, Mou, how are you?"

"I'm good." But then I said, "We should hang out sometime."

"Yea, that would be fun!"

It was only a few days later, when I was drinking Strawberry Hill with my girl gang from the sixth floor, that I got up the nerve to go and bug Sally. I was so curious. Is it true what Harriet had said?

I told my girls that I would be right back. I grabbed what was left of one of the open bottles and I started to leave.

"Where are you going?"

"I'm going to invite my friend Sally to join us."

I stumbled down the stairs to the 5th floor and knocked on Sally and Harriet's door. No answer. I knocked again, although I knew if someone was home they would've opened the door by now. Those dorm rooms were awfully small.

No answer. I started to turn around to walk back up the stairs when I saw someone walking towards me from the other direction. She spotted me immediately.

"Hey, Mou!"

"Oh hey, Sally! I was just coming down to see if you wanted to come join us upstairs - me and some of the girls are having drinks."

"Yea, sure! Let me just drop this stuff off at my room." She motioned to the groceries in her hand.

I handed her some of my Strawberry Hill as she organized some things in her room.

"Strawberry Hill?" She laughed as she unpacked her groceries. "Look what I got?" She showed me a 6-pack of wine coolers she had just bought.

"Great!"

We both started laughing and the night began.

It wasn't too long before I asked the question I was dying to know. We were still in her room. Sally was taking her sweet time, so I got comfortable and settled in on her dorm bed. (The dorms were small, shared rooms, so it was common that beds also doubled as guest seating.)

"Hey, so Sally," I paused, then continued, "Harriet told me something about you." I knew that sounded so gossipy, but at least I was asking her to her face and not spreading rumors around town.

Sally looked over at me with a sly smile on her face as though she knew where this was going, or maybe she also felt the phrasing was gossipy.

"Yes?" she asked.

"Harriet told me that you have a girlfriend. Is that true?"

Sally continued doing what she was doing - which was who knows what... like organizing her groceries still?! - and kept her back turned to me for what seemed like the longest minute ever.

Then, she finally turned around. She regained her composure and she said, "Yes," she pursed her lips. "What Harriet said is true. I do have a girlfriend." She seemed defensive, on guard, and I immediately knew the feeling.

I quickly jumped in and said, "I dated a couple girls too." I didn't want Harriet to get in trouble so I followed it up with, "Harriet knows some of my friends, that's how the topic came up."

Sally seemed perplexed. I think she thought I was hitting on her. So I made a few more clarifications.

"I guess I identify as bi. How about you?"

She was quiet and nodded.

"Yea, I guess so."

"It's hard to meet girls who are bi and cool."

She started to warm up. "Yeah, I know what you mean."

She took a sip of her drink, looked at herself in the mirror and said, "Let's go upstairs."

She was finally ready.

On our way up the stairs, we bumped into several friends and acquaintances. We both had been living in the dorms for about 2 weeks at this point and everyone was starting to become familiar faces.

"I need to go to the bathroom," Sally said then pivoted towards the bathroom as we walked by the one on the 6th floor. At this point we were both buzzing pretty hard.

"Come with," she said, using her hand to gesture.

The next thing you know Sally and I were sitting on the shower floor just talking about our lives. Turns out we had more things in common than just dating women. We knew some of the same people, listened to the same music, went to the same underground nightclubs (there were 3 well-known ones across the 3 counties) and had similar tastes in friends and fashion.

At some point our other friends found us in the bathroom, but by this point Sally and I were drunk.

"There you are!"

"Hey, Sally!"

"What are you guys doing?"

Sally and I joined the others, and the night went on like so many other nights in the dorms. Late nights with lots of friends.

Sally and I kept our sexual identity a secret from our dorm friends. We would sneak off into the night and go to the local lesbian bars. We started learning who some of the other lesbians were in the dorms. For me, it was an exciting time and all I wanted was to go to the lesbian clubs and bars to meet more queer women. Sally was my wing woman, and I hers. People at the bars thought we were a couple, but that was the furthest thing from the truth.

Sally had a girlfriend who still lived in the suburb she came from, and they were "working things out." Sally's ex-girlfriend was also still in the picture, very much still in love with Sally and also had a fling with Sally's current girlfriend. These similarities in our first lesbian triadic relationships were uncanny also and this made our friendship that much stronger. We were both coming out and having such similar and parallel experiences.

One particular night, Sally and I got ahold of some magic mushrooms and decided to go out on the town. It was a cold and rainy night and not much was going on in the Castro District, our default go-to spot. It was the gay part of town and we always felt at home just walking around there. Maybe we'd stop in to get a coffee. Maybe we'd go to a bar. That night after much giggling and walking around in the rain, we decided it was time to head home, so we laughed as we took our mushroom-laced, rain-soaked selves down to the Castro train station. We were chatting away and waiting for the train as we often did when we spotted a lone bumper sticker on the wall.

The sticker said, "Straight Poop." Sally and I both read it aloud. "STRAIGHT. POOP."

Silence. And then the a-ha moment. This was the phrase I had been looking for, that summed up our entire coming out experience. Straight Poop. The existence of learning to live in a heterosexual world that didn't accept nor understand us. There it was. Straight Poop.

That night we knew what we had to do. We could no longer hide.

The M train dropped us off at the corner of Holloway and we walked across campus in the rain, contemplating what we just learned about ourselves and life. We finally knew who we were and we could see everything so clearly.

We got back to the dorms and we went straight up to the 6th floor. Our gang of girls were all there hanging out in the usual dorm room they hung out in.

It was raining, so everyone was in for the night.

Sally and I walked in and we were quickly welcomed.

"Hey, Sally!"

"Hey, Mou!"

"Hey guys."

"Where have you been?"

"Were you guys out?"

It was time to come clean.

That night we finally let the girls know our story. How we met, and where we had been going.

"We're bi."

"We've been going to the girl clubs."

And, we got all kinds of reactions. All good reactions.

"That's cool."

"Really? You were afraid to tell us?!?"

"I kind of had a feeling."

"Awesome."

"Did you meet anyone yet?"

And hugs, lots of hugs, smiles, laughter and support.

And then it was business as usual.

"Pass me the wine cooler."

We were all back chatting about mid-terms and music and boys and now girls, too.

You would think coming out would get easier the more you do it, but the truth is coming out never gets easier. The trauma can come up every single time. You never know what kind of response you will get. Sometimes you get re-traumatized which can make things harder down the road. And sometimes you get lucky and have a corrective emotional experience. The people who accept you for who you are, make you stronger, which can in turn maybe reduce the effects of trauma.

❧ Chapter 12 ☙

You Never Know...
(Who Needs to Hear This?)
1991

When Bonnie found out I was bisexual she immediately developed a crush on me. We had been friends in high school, and she met me after I had broken up with Cleo. Somehow, she didn't get the memo about my sexuality until I was well into my first year at SFSU. It wasn't premeditated nor thought out. It was easy. I had hidden my bisexuality from Bonnie.

I was scared to tell Bonnie that I had dated women. Maybe I assumed she already knew.

Bonnie grew up in the suburbs like me. She had a crush on all my male buddies, many of whom were bi and/or gay themselves. She was clearly into boys. Everyone thought Bonnie was pretty. She was my height with black shiny hair. I always assumed she was straight.

One afternoon, I was picking Bonnie up from her house. Our families lived close to each other. It was the summer after my senior year. I would be heading off to college in the city soon. Bonnie was a year younger than me, so she still lived at home and had another year of school left.

I drove over the hill to meet Bonnie at her house in the suburban landscape where we grew up. Her family lived in a neighborhood with big houses, McMansions of the 1980's which colored the way we grew up.

Bonnie's mother was sweet like apple pie. Well-read, educated, white. Their house was quite big. Beautiful manicured front yard, complete with water fountain. Short driveway, with three European cars parked in the driveway. Their backyard was covered with shade from big fruit trees, with beautiful Roman statues and lots of roses. I loved the roses.

It was a sunny day, and I was relaxing in the backyard with Bonnie's mom, sipping lemonade. "Bonnie will be right down," she said as she let me in. "You can sit in the shade and wait for her." She led me through the den, through the kitchen and into the peaceful backyard. The smell of roses filled the air, while Buster their little miniature poodle nipped at my heels. I walked around in the yard. I could hear Bonnie's mom say, "Bonnie, hurry up and get dressed. You're being rude to your guest." Her voice neared and I heard the screen door slide open. "Here you go, dear. I don't know what is taking Bonnie so long." She placed a tall glass of what looked like iced lemonade on a coaster as I approached the table.

I sat down and listened to the birds chirping. Bonnie's mother began watering plants when Bonnie came running in. Her hair was chopped hanging in uneven strands everywhere and Bonnie was completely naked.

"Bonnie, put some clothes on." Her mother gasped in horror.

Bonnie yelled something incoherent at her mom. She was frantic. "Mou, don't listen to her."

I was stunned. What was going on here? "Are you ready?"

But, I was fascinated by the drama. I was getting an inside

peek of life at Bonnie's. "Mom, you don't know anything. Just leave me alone." Bonnie was yelling. Her mom still pleading with her to get dressed.

I was perplexed. I knew Bonnie had two older brothers. And, her parents were still married. At 5 feet tall with long cascading hair covering her breasts, she looked like a gothic queen from the sci fi movies. Yes, this felt like a sexual thing, although I could be wrong. Was this something being thrown in her mother's face? What had her mother done?

"Oh, get over it, Mother." Bonnie went into the kitchen and poured herself a tall glass of lemonade and laid down on the couch. Ass cheeks hanging out, breasts covered by her hair, even I was uncomfortable. In my house we were always covered up. Nude Bonnie and her mother argued back and forth for a few minutes, about something I couldn't figure out. Finally, I said, "Bonnie, are we still going?" Bonnie did not answer. Her mother tried telling me that Bonnie was not up for it.

Bonnie interrupted her and said, "I am going!"

I started to get up to leave. "No," Bonnie yelled at her mom. But she didn't move.

I was caught in some weird mother-daughter fight where the daughter, my friend Bonnie, was storming around the house naked. I had no idea what I had walked into.

I got up and started gathering my belongings. "Give me a call when you're ready."

Bonnie just lay there exasperated on the couch.

I scurried out of the house, into my car, and down the road as fast as I could.

We never did go out that night. Several weeks later I would be moving to San Francisco and my whole life and friend group would drastically change.

By the time she found out about my sexuality, Bonnie and I had stopped hanging out as much. I was deeply steeped in my lesbian world.

I came home for the summer, right after my first year of college. That was the only time I would do that. I still kept my job in San Francisco working at Crabtree and Evelyn, the soap store, so I was traveling to San Francisco several times during the week.

I was still friends with Cleo, my ex from high school. We hung out sometimes, but it was awkward. She had a new girlfriend, and so did I, but her residual anger with me still lingered, and would linger for the rest of our lives. In her mind, I was an opportunist and instigator.

"You play mind games," she would say. And, in my mind, she was playing the victim. Tomato, tomah-to. I guess. We would never reconcile this. But this particular day, I swung by her place on my way from work. Her was apartment in the suburbs, where she lived comfortably with her new girlfriend.

Cleo immediately launched in, "She was crying tears because she likes you," Cleo said while laughing in between her words. "Hahaha." Cleo was being simultaneously rude and supportive, if that's possible. "Can you believe it, Mou, Bonnie!? She likes you! She was crying tears over you." As if it would never be possible for a pretty suburban girl to like someone like me. Brown. And I assumed she meant unattractive.

I wasn't surprised. This felt typical and suspiciously convenient. I was considered a femme, a lipstick lesbian. Lipstick lesbians are often the gateway to the queer world. We look straight enough, which is safe. Read: we don't rock the boat, making it easy for others to experiment, and come out if it "worked."

Suddenly, I was given news that one of the prettiest girls in our old friend group liked me and I was expected to jump?

Bonnie wasn't the type of girl I was interested in.

I didn't care for what the male gaze liked. I personally was into more masc or masculine presenting folks who weren't exploring their sexuality for the first time.

I was simultaneously happy though to hear that Bonnie could now embrace the sexual fluidity inside of herself, even if we weren't meant to be together. I felt that in a way I had at least helped someone acknowledge something else existed inside of them.

Assumptions are the hardest part of embracing your fluidity. Today, there is more wiggle room, but we still grapple with these ideas of beauty, of desire, and what a fluid, bisexual or queer person is supposed to look like.

Bonnie knew her beauty appealed to the male gaze, and sometimes she flaunted it.

I was flattered by Bonnie's attraction to me on the one hand because it felt good to learn that she accepted my sexuality. But I was simultaneously confused by it. Her attraction felt sudden and in direct response to learning I was bi. Simple acceptance or rejection was easier. Things were more complicated when coming out created attraction. I guess it made the acceptance feel conditional.

On the other hand, I knew that bisexual exploration is a common desire for women. Maybe I was a safe harbor for that exploration with my long hair and feminine looks. Maybe she didn't know any other way or better yet, maybe she didn't know any people with whom she could come out or explore her sexuality. It was a lot of responsibility for 19-year-old me to wrap my head around. It wasn't something I really wanted to be a part of.

Bonnie and I stayed friends after that, but the weight of the information about her crush created a wedge and eventually we drifted apart.

ဆ Chapter 13 ၼ

Slutting Around Is Radical
1991

One might say my popularity in San Francisco went to my head. I don't think of myself as the vengeful type, but I was definitely out to change the narrative. I was angry at the [heteronormative] girls who put looks and boys ahead of sisterhood and friendship. I really hated how some (many) girls would look you up and down, checking to see if your outfit, body type, hairstyle, jewelry and accessories all fit into some mold of something acceptable (this was a sign of the hetero "normative" ones who had bought into capitalism, the patriarchy, and toxic masculinity, had drank the Kool-Aid, so to speak.) Acceptable to who? I was always feeling judged for not being feminine enough, pretty enough, dainty enough. However, I knew who they were trying to impress. Succumbing to the socially acceptable ways of presenting oneself.

Yea, I was cynical, and angry.

From a young age, girls in our society are taught to please the male gaze. But by the time it enters our awareness, we have been so conditioned by the macro culture, which in the United States is a predominantly patriarchal, predominantly Christian, mostly heteronormative purview, that we think this idea of beauty is obvious, normal, or worse, we don't even question it.

What is deemed attractive and a standard that is upheld by women and men alike in our society could be argued is from a male gaze, and is quite childlike in its nature and look. Thin is revered. Women who have little to no curves, almost like children or little boys, are deemed the most attractive in our society. Straight hair that is blown out and smooth. Again, like a young child's. These are the things that stood out to me growing up in the suburbs. And, as I have gotten older I see how hard this is to achieve and maintain. One only needs to open the pages of any fashion or glamour magazine to see the amount of things they try to sell women to look young.

As a brown-skinned, black curly-haired girl growing up in a land that revered blonde-haired thin white women, I was not used to getting a lot of attention. So, when I began getting attention for the first time, I began getting my confidence. It was really validating to get attention. For the first time in my life, I felt seen.

I was also living alone for the first time, albeit on campus, and on one particular night my multicultural girl dorm gang – group of females who were my main group that first year in the dorms (who reminded me a lot of my diverse little-girl gang I'd long since forgotten about from 5th grade in Oak Ridge) went out on the town.

The girls and I had decided to go to a local club, but it was almost midnight, and we knew not to expect much being that it was also a Wednesday night.

We ended up at a bar where I bumped into some guys who knew me from the underage club scene I had been frequenting since I was 16. My worlds were colliding.

My worlds would collide quite often. In fact, there was a lot of overlap so it was never surprising. The only difference was that now I lived in San Francisco proper and was a few years older. And more confident.

I didn't know Roger very well. I only knew that he dated Mollye, a tight knit friend of Bonnie's. In fact, I would not have recognized him unless he hadn't said something to me first.

"Hey, Mou," I heard someone say. I wasn't surprised at that either. I worked the clubs, so this knowing people from my current life was pretty normal. But, as I turned around, the face looking at me was not very familiar and neither was the voice. "Hey, Mou, what's up? It's Roger." I must have looked confused. Where did I know him from. But before I could ask, he stuttered, "Um... Mollye's boyfriend."

"Oh, heyyyy, Roger," I said, putting him at ease with my comforting style. "How are you?" I leaned in for a hug, the normal thing to do among friends.

Roger was known to be good looking, and there was always a surprise when people learned he dated Mollye, which I didn't understand. Mollye was attractive and had a nice style. I didn't know her well, but she seemed very nice, albeit somewhat quiet. One thing I did pick up from Mollye and her friends was that quiet judgment girls often gave other girls. I got it from most girls. I always chalked it up to heteronormativity and toxic masculinity, but of course it could've been something else altogether, like the color of my skin. But, of course, I could never voice this feeling I had. It was the 1980's. It wasn't commonplace to talk about these issues, especially not in the suburbs.

In fact, oppressed groups are often told they are overreacting, being hypersensitive, imagining it and/or being paranoid. That's in fact a form of gaslighting.

In San Francisco in the 1990's, not many talked about systemic injustices. But so many of us could feel it. Many live within the rules of society, and this was what I was unknowingly fighting all along and what I was simultaneously learning more and more about and waking up to, at my university.

Pretty soon my girls and his guys were all hanging around just having a fun time. We were drinking, goofing around, chit-chatting.

Roger was flirting with me, and it was fine. I was enjoying the attention. The funny thing is I was the opposite of Mollye. Where she was feminine and soft spoken, I was rough and tumble. I was loud and brash about my drug use, my sexuality. She was demure and discerning. That night especially I felt free from the stifling femininity and rules many heterosexual girls felt they had to obey, which I finally knew I no longer would nor feel I needed to obey.

Eventually the bar closed and everyone decided to take the party back to the dorms where more drinking continued. I was someone they wanted to follow. He said that he and Mollye had broken up. I had no reason not to believe him. I was embracing and feeling the power in my queer sexuality.

Later the news spread like wildfire. I had slept with Mollye's boyfriend. What kind of a person would do that? I did it because I could.

In the heteronormative world, the other woman is to blame. Women blame each other. No one looks at the man involved. I'm curious, why is the man not to blame? No one even looked at Roger. Why was it suddenly something I did?

Despite being blamed, and the sex not even being good, there was something more to this story. There was some redemption. I was kind of smiling inside. What I did felt good. Was this some sort of revenge? To be able to get back at the straight girls? Maybe so... I was getting way more attention these days in San Francisco than I had ever experienced, and I took it upon myself to do something, because I could. But I felt empowered and disconnected from the stories and voices on the other side. In my heart I knew, I was not to blame.

But there was more to it. I was a single woman coming into my own. And being in the wild west of what we now label as queer, kink and ethical non-monogamy, I was privy to lifestyles and new relationship rules that were more intuitive, forgiving, and real, rules the heteronormative world was missing out on!

I wanted to teach the hetero world a lesson, but more so I wanted to inspire them and educate them about sexual freedom, about autonomy, owning our bodies and doing what feels good, about not playing into the rules of the patriarchy, like ownership and possession, jealousy and assumed exclusivity, and about how toxic masculinity and the patriarchy had taken freedoms and so much more away from us.

Yep. I was here, I had finally arrived. I was going to show them that being unabashedly yourself could be attractive too. We needn't follow the rules of normative culture. And furthermore, I was going to show the world that all these unspoken rules, for women and men, to live in the straight and narrow, it certainly screwed me, and it was screwing them, too.

౿ Chapter 14 ౷

U of L
(Read: Maybe This Monogamy
Thing Isn't Working for Me)
1993

As the M Ocean View barreled outbound through the fog over Twin Peaks and out towards Lakeside and Balboa Park, I looked around and noticed who was riding with me. College students with their book bags, holding their coffee, reading their books. I was in my typical U of L (San Francisco State University was affectionately dubbed by the locals as University of Lesbians or U of L) "uniform," as one professor pointed out that we all have uniforms. Students, teachers, etc. Mine was always the same, except for that short stint when I was working at the bank and had to come straight to class. I wasn't allowed to wear jeans at the bank, so I'd wear slacks, black oxfords with the shoelaces and vintage jackets from the thrift store. I tried to keep it retro even though I was working somewhere corporate and stuffy.

But today I had on my real uniform and favorite attire: lace up black Dr. Martens boots, faded Levi jeans and a vintage leather jacket. It was right after I had quit my job at the bank, and I was excited to get back into a more creative vibe. These clothes represented that. Working at a bank left me stifled, rigid. College was supposed to be about me. This was supposed to be my time, learning, and cultivating myself as a creative and critical thinker, reading literature and true histories of Black Americans, of suffragettes, and Stonewall, the things that weren't being taught in American public schools back then. Drinking coffee on the grass under a tree, I had music playing in my headphones. Like always. Headphones were a must because they would play the bands, mixtapes, and artists, female fronted, independent, rock n roll, protest singers, electronica and Grrrl rock, that were the soundtracks to my life then.

San Francisco State University was known as a "commuter school." That's what I was told before I started going there. What this meant mostly was that people didn't live on campus, nor even near the campus. Most people commute to the campus. From other parts of the city and from other parts of the Bay Area too. I wanted the college experience, so my first year, I lived on campus.

The campus is situated on Holloway Avenue on the southside past the city, south of the hustle and bustle, past the Sunset District and further out, close to a lake just inland from the ocean. It's a damp, dark and predominantly gray area of the city, and sunshine is a rarer occurrence here, as the area is often covered in marine layer. This gloom feeds the romanticism of a northern academic town.

Fall was my favorite time of year to be in school. I got my coffee, walked through the quad and then began getting settled in the library. I preferred a window seat so I could people-watch. The window overlooked the quad area.

I imagined people's lives, loves and academic pursuits. Sometimes I would study, but daydreaming is what got me through school.

Every now and again I would see an interracial lesbian couple. They wore jeans, black coats, beanies and even an occasional beret. One of them wrote poetry, I was told.

I sat and recalled my lesbian teacher from my first year at SFSU, my first semester in fact. My friend George was in my class. George was a gay boy who I knew from before coming to SFSU. He had dated a good friend of mine. She inspired us to write stories about our histories. George wrote a great story about growing up gay. I think I wrote my story about being a feminist and hating thin culture, but she wanted me to write about the fact that the Barbie in my story was blonde. She wanted me to write about my experience as a non-white person, as a brown person. But I wasn't ready.

I was ready to dismantle the patriarchy, though. The fact that I so readily embraced lesbianism was my signal to myself that I wanted to fight closed-mindedness, but I didn't know that was about oppression on a grand scale. My mind knew I didn't want anything of the traditional sense. No nuclear family, no kids, no 9 to 5. I had a renegade heart; this I knew and those early years in San Francisco I craved acceptance. I needed to find my tribe so I could thrive. Relationships were the easiest thing. One-on-one relationships were easier to cultivate than finding a large group of friends.

Christa and I would study together. But she wasn't studying Psychology like she had before. She left her old life behind to come to San Francisco, but she never did go back to school. She would occasionally meet me at the library after work and on weekends.

On weekends we would travel to other libraries to study. UCSF's library was beautiful, so we went there sometimes. It's located in the upper Haight Ashbury area, so it was surrounded by lots of life. Not to mention the library itself had mahogany tables and was all around beautiful. The school sat on a hill, so there were some lovely views as well. This fed my romantic, academic dreams. I would imagine the literary students, the beat writers all converging here in San Francisco. But I was starting to get bored. All study and living in my head was no fun and was starting to get old.

My relationship was too comfortable. She loved me and doted on me. And the overwhelming loneliness I felt in prior years was squelched during our 4-year relationship.

We lived in a small apartment in the mission, on an adorable street in a hip part of town. I needed to get out of the house. If I could have had it my way, I would be doing something a little more creative, fun even, but going to the library gave me purpose, and my goal was to do well in school. Being with her kept me in line and out of trouble. But I was ready for a change.

The day we met I was 19. I had just finished my first year at San Francisco State University and was working at the British Soap and Perfume Store. I had moved home to the suburbs but was driving into SF several times a week for work.

It was a Saturday and the store was traditionally busy on Saturdays as it was located in a popular tourist location. Christa walked in at some point, but the store was so busy I had not had a chance to acknowledge her just yet. Finally the store quieted down for a moment and I noticed her thumbing through a book.

"Hello," I said, "anything I can help you with today?"

She looked up from her book. And with nary a shift in her facial expression she said calmly and matter-of-factly, "Hi, Mou."

"Oh hey," I said, thinking maybe this was a friend from high school. I couldn't quite place her face yet.

"I'm Christa. I'm a friend of Jade's. I'm just visiting for the summer."

A friend of Jade's? Jade and I hooked up in the dorms a few times, but she did not want to have anything to do with me beyond that.

"Oh cool! Nice to meet you," I said. At that moment, luckily some new patrons walked in, and I was able to walk away from Christa, if only momentarily to help the other customers.

Did Jade send her? What did she want? My heart had taken a few months to get over Jade so I was unsure why she would be sending her friends around now.

As I was finished talking with the customers, Christa came back over and asked, "Do you get a break soon?"

"Sure, I can take a break in a few."

I saw my studious co-worker sitting out in the courtyard reading and I hollered to her out the window, "Hey, Lara, I'm ready for a break whenever you are."

Lara was easy going, and since there were no managers with us on Saturdays we took breaks whenever we needed, relying on the other to operate the small store in our absence.

Christa and I walked around the square and she told me she was a lesbian and was interested in moving here to San Francisco, as she'd heard there were many gay women here.

"I just need to get out of Dallas. It's so straight."

"Yes, I can totally imagine."

"Do you have a girlfriend?" she asked. She was so serious and barely showed any emotion. Later I would find out she was just nervous.

"Nope," I said.

"Do you want to go out later?"

"Yes. Yes, I do."

We went out that night. She claimed that she saw my photo and took one look at me and was hooked, and then came out to San Francisco to find me, or someone like me. Queer. Femme.

Christa on the other hand was a few inches shorter than me, and she had more masc-presenting appearance. Short beach blonde hair, athletic, sporty and what many would call "Tomboy."

We then spent the rest of the summer together, inseparable. And I blossomed sexually. I had my first partnered orgasm and I finally learned how to insert a tampon. I was learning about my body in ways I may never have with a man.

When the fall came, she had to go back home to finish out the semester and then her plan was to transfer to San Francisco State.

My life changed that year. I had spent my first year at SFSU going to nightclubs, hooking up with girls and boys and failing my classes. My second year, I was in a relationship with Christa. I got straight A's, stopped going to clubs, and stopped going out. I buckled down and got serious. For the first time ever, I got my life on track and together.

Every morning I would get up early and run laps on the track at school. After school I went to work at the perfumery and then after work I came home to share a good night call with Christa.

"How was your day?"

"Good. How was yours?"

"I miss you."

"I miss you too."

When Christa finally moved back to SF after tying up all her loose ends at school, we moved in together and did almost everything together.

One year turned to two years turned to three years and the boredom was increasing. It was easy to cocoon with Christa, but together we weren't doing anything revolutionary, and the great sex had died within the first year or so. I began to feel restless in the relationship.

One day I sat in the library, trying to study, and wondered, *Is it time to break up?*

Christa was working at a job that was so different from my academic world. She had moved out here to transfer but was having difficulty getting those credits transferred.

But why would you break up with someone who just worships the ground you walk on?

I tried to study. But my mind kept wandering.

A lot of the women (and men) in the queer and LGBT community in San Francisco were participating in sexually fluid *and* relationally fluid lifestyles. I wanted to explore non-monogamy with Christa but had no idea how to bring it up to her. I wanted to join the ranks of creative lesbians living their best lives, but I was stuck. I didn't think she'd go for it anyway.

I began to feel resentful in my relationship.

This morning before we had left the house, she had asked, "What were you and Lynda doing last night so late?"

She was often jealous of my closest girlfriends, Lynda and Lucia.

"Nothing, just hanging out, gossiping, trying on clothes," I said casually, as I put my head back down and continued packing my backpack. I had lots of close relationships with other people. Intimate, but not physically intimate, nor even romantic. I never harbored delusions that one person could fulfill all my emotional needs. As a self-identified extrovert, I needed a lot of mental stimulation. I needed my friends.

She huffed and puffed and rolled her eyes and said, "But you did that last week, too."

She came over and put her arm around me.

"Last week we went to The Café," I said, pushing her off me.

The Café was a popular gay and lesbian bar in the heart of The Castro where we would often go after class for a quick drink, and it was a place where we spent many a drunken night.

"What were you guys doing there?" Now she started to sound accusatory. Angry even.

"What is with the 20 questions?" I snapped back. This was a typical conversation these days. She was mostly sweet but sometimes these insinuations would seep out. She was opinionated about my friends. I was defensive. But we both kept it going as cordially as we could. We were in a committed monogamous relationship, after all.

The irony is that in my life I would find myself here so many times. Long-term relationships that grow stale. Jealous partners who just feel left out. Monogamy that turns into monotony and chokes us while we sleep. We love security, until it turns to suffocation.

Truth be told, the previous week Nell, a sexy tall androgynous woman with short brown hair and glasses, had started flirting with me at The Café. Though I hadn't done anything "wrong," in monogamous terms, meaning nothing physical, in my heart I knew I had developed a little crush on Nell. And I was "guilty" of flirting and essentially breaking the biggest unspoken assumption in monogamy, that you should only be attracted to your partner. A faulty idea which goes completely against our true human and sexual nature. Furthermore, I knew that this piece of information would only validate Christa's already vulnerable sense of security in us. Another malady of monogamy is to just accept this type of codependency. We "read our partner's mind," in this sense. We don't talk about crushes, feelings for others, attractions. That is taboo in monogamy. And it was in our relationship too. Now, I am not saying you should willfully tell your partner how hot you think someone else is to hurt them, but you can set some parameters around honest discussion, and manage expectations within the relationship, by acknowledging this truth.

I twirled my pencil as I watched Christa reading her book. Right then she looked up and smiled at me.

"Hey do you wanna get outta here?" I asked. "I think I might be getting hungry."

"Sure!" She got up and started packing up.

As we were leaving the library, I spotted Nell on campus. There she was just right in front of the library. My heart skipped a beat, and immediately I was annoyed that I was with Christa. I felt like I was with my mom. (*Cue the psychobabble about how we often create relationships that mimic our families of origin.)

Christa knew Nell from the scene but didn't think much of her. She had negative opinions about many lesbians. They didn't meet her aesthetic standards. She liked the femmes.

Nell, on the other hand, studied at U of L too, majoring in Foreign Policy.

Nell didn't see me. She was talking to a friend. I started walking over, with Christa in tow, when Nell looked up. I waved and said, "Hi."

Nell stopped talking to her friend and gave a warm smile and said, "Hey!"

She gave me a tight and sensual hug and then turned and introduced us to her friend.

"You remember Christa?" I asked.

"Sure!" Nell smiled at Christa and shook her hand. Shook her hand?! I just knew this was going to raise Christa's suspicions.

"We're getting ready for the Clinic fundraiser, what are you two up to?"

"Oh just studying," I said.

Nell was busy doing socially important work that mattered. I was boring. I studied and in my spare time I went to the bars. I was simple. I was boring.

"Cool, well see you later."

"Bye."

"Nice to see you again."

We walked off then, but my heart was heavy. I just wanted to go back and say, "Hey, can I help?" or, "What are you doing later? Let's hang out."

I wanted so desperately to be pulled out of the drudgery that was my life. I felt like I was missing out big time.

Non-monogamy, age and understanding codependency has taught me to say what you want to say, and to say it in front of your partners. Women are taught to protect other's feelings. It's a form of oppression.

A few weeks later, I would be hanging out at the Café with some friends. I managed to get out, alone. This was often the case if it was after class. Nell was also there. We were drinking and flirting, having a good time.

At some point Nell said, "We should have a threesome," she pointed to another girl–and me. "Totally," the other girl exclaimed.

"Hell yes, I would."

This would not be my first non-monogamous experience.

I had hooked up in a group setting on molly a few times prior.

Of course, I didn't want to cheat. I would have to talk to Christa about our relationship. Something was going to have to give. But I was scared.

I was not ready to jeopardize the safety of our monogamous relationship.

Instead of talking to Christa when I got home, I wrote about it in my journal. I wanted to bond and talk openly with Christa. She was my best friend after all, but I was finding it so hard to focus. I was excited for the possibilities and scared of how Christa would respond. That night I left it alone. It was just so easy to surrender to the safety of our twosome.

The next day when I came home from school, Christa was crying. She had read my journal. In my journal I made no mention of ethical non-monogamy and having a discussion with Christa, I just talked about my excitement and desire for Nell, and having a threesome with Nell. It was all about Nell.

Whether Christa felt my distance and had a hunch, or had been doing it all along, journal reading is a violation in and of itself. It leads to a loss of trust and there was no way in hell Christa would agree to try ethical non-monogamy, not after this. In that moment, we lost that trust. My journal was my therapy. A place to work out thoughts, make plans. For Christa, it was a place for me to harbor secrecy and dishonesty. I hid my feelings for Nell and the fact that I wanted to be with someone else, at all. I had never spoken up about ethical non-monogamy. Had I brought it up sooner and made her feel truly safe by talking about commitment instead of love, I may have created some healthier, more realistic expectations in our relationship. Instead, we tell each other this lie in relationships, *I love you and only you forever.*

That was the beginning of the end. Looking back, we were young. I had no role models for healthy same sex, non-monogamy. I was winging it. Monogamy and cheating were the only frames that I really knew about. Heteronormativity. And it pretty much shaped everything.

Today, I believe you can have the things you want in relationships. Well, almost everything. But you will never know unless you ask, talk, and plant seeds. Managing expectations when you get into a relationship is great, but what if you don't know? We can't expect to know what will come up in our relationships as we grow, change and evolve. So, we get clear about our needs first. Yes, journaling is an excellent way of doing so. Your journal is a private space to explore ideas. Nothing in your journal is written in stone. Tell your partner that your journal is off limits, for this reason alone. It's dangerous, unthought-out territory. If a partner doesn't like you to have even that amount of privacy, you have an issue on your hands. Trust is a two-way street.

A therapist is great, too. A place to process your thoughts. When you are ready to start talking to your partner about "taboo" topics, such as attraction to others outside of your couple bubble, or anything that goes against our assumptions about monogamy, I always suggest going slow and planting seeds. Let them get used to the ideas you have before bombarding them. That's just a suggestion. You can bombard them too. Either way, I recommend honesty. If your partner is closed off by non-monogamous ideas, you need this information as soon as possible. This will help you make your decisions. This helps to also give them the information. They might change their mind, too.

Also, relationships could focus on the commitment we make to each other. *I commit to put you first today,* instead of, *I love you forever,* which sets up clear expectations and are based in reality, not fantasy and fairy tale.

Bottom line is to keep an open mind, go slow, be patient, and most of all, be honest. Remember, it's not always going to be easy being this radically honest. Especially in a culture that often feels like it values monogamy and cheating over radical honesty.

❧ Chapter 15 ☙

My Intro to Non-Monogamy (Read: "Why Wasn't I Good Enough?") 1994-1995

I walked away from my last relationship ready to embrace my creativity in so many ways, including my sexuality.

I knew who I needed to be around. They were creative. They were artsy. They were poets and musicians and painters and writers. They were wild. They wore leather. They were tattooed. They were queer. They rode motorcycles or bicycles. They owned venues and lived in warehouses, or in houses with gardens, or in vans. I thought that dating Nell might be a start in the right direction.

I let Nell walk all over me. I mean, I really loved the idea of non-monogamy, especially after my last stifling relationship. I loved the idea, but I didn't know the rules. And I didn't know what to ask.

The running story ended up being that I wasn't good enough.

I was guilty, too, of not openly communicating my feelings, expressing my concerns, wants, desires. I went along with it. I had been conditioned in the monogamous community. And, had I known the rules of ethical non-monogamy, then I might have had more success.

"We can sleep with other people one time only. After that we become attached. We are more likely to become emotionally involved," Nell said matter-of-factly. She knew what she wanted. And, she knew the truth about our sexual selves and bodies. She also knew the rules of ethical non-monogamy. Or, at least, to the newbie lay person, myself, it just made so much sense. I really loved the idea. And, I knew in my gut this was so good for us, and so healthy. But aside from this one statement rule, we never discussed anything beyond it.

"If that happens, we need to tell each other."

"I like that." It felt honest. At the time.

I wanted honesty. And, the ability to go out, flirt with other people, possibly even hook up without having to worry about how my partner felt was so freeing. What I didn't realize is the first part of the one-fuck rule, also supported "don't ask, don't tell."

"Don't ask, don't tell," was a term I became familiar with in ethical non-monogamy, but it really came to be because the military didn't want gay people to come out. "Don't ask, don't tell," supports secrecy under the guise of supporting privacy. If you are a straight person, you may be asking yourself what the difference is? Isn't privacy good? Yes, of course, privacy is good. What we do behind closed doors should be private. But the LGBT communities don't need privacy when it comes to equal rights. The right to marry someone of the same gender. The right to hold hands with their partner in the street. The queer community needs more visibility and "don't ask, don't tell" is a form of erasure, keeping gay people hidden away from public view, in the closet forever, under the guise of privacy.

We spent a lovely evening together that night. Nell cooked pasta and we had sex. She was an incredible lover. She was a top, and she knew what she was doing. She always had the lube, the sex toys ready by the bed, and often she had a plan. She knew what she wanted the sex to look like. I got to enjoy the ride. I became a full-on bottom in this relationship. No pressure to be anything else.

As a psychotherapist specializing in sex and kink, one thing I have learned about dominance and submission that has really rung true for me is the fact that our sexual language often complements who we are. By day an achiever, a leader, a CEO, in bed may prefer to be more submissive, a bottom, a pillow princess. The desire is to completely surrender.

With Nell I continued to explore the edges of my sexuality.

I walked home that morning feeling mostly great. But once at home, the loneliness would seep in. The anxiety of dating Nell was always there, simmering under my skin. I didn't feel safe and secure in the relationship. And, I didn't know that I could openly talk about it. I often wondered later however, was I really inexperienced or did I feel something else, for example, if I brought it up that she might dismiss my concerns? I like to remember that we often act or don't act, not because we don't know we can but because we don't think we can, we don't feel we have room or permission.

Today, I know the insecurity did not stem from our "open relationship," per se. Knowing how to navigate ethical monogamy takes time, and understanding is not necessarily easy, and communication is key.

My gut told me that Nell wanted to avoid communication. Her general rule that required two fucks before you would open up a conversation left a lot of uncommunicated gray area. As a therapist today, I certainly would not recommend this to partners who I work with and coach. It's a personal choice of course, but communication is the cornerstone of healthy non-monogamy.

I lived in a state of anxiety. We didn't live together. And, I had no idea what she was up to when we were apart, which was a lot of the time. I know I could have been sowing my own oats. I wanted to. And, I was too distracted to do so.

We weren't committed. Not in the monogamous sense. That was the bottom line. According to our label and agreement we were dating and open, but the overnights and time we spent together spelled relationship to me. It was confusing. We were dating and open. Fair enough. I didn't ask her for more communication. I convinced myself that it was too early in the relationship for that. I waited around for her. When she would call me and want to spend time with me, it validated my worth. In my heart I believed I valued myself more, but by accepting that relationship as it was, without conversations about my feelings, my actions spoke louder than my words. The message was loud and clear. I did not think I was good enough.

This internal message had to do with my work as an artist more than anything else. Creativity and art were tied up with these women during these years.

"You're so simple," Nell exclaimed one night. It was a jab. And it hurt. But I knew she was right. I didn't have much else going on except for school, and once I graduated I got a job. I wanted to play music but I had no idea where to start, and even if I did put myself out there I was unprepared. I had yet to write a song.

I waited for her to take me out, introduce me to people. I was an outsider looking in. I was out of my league. Or, so I believed.

I finally left that relationship when I had enough. Of the cheating. (Yes, the one-fuck rule eventually led to betrayal, something that happens even in "open relationships.") I had had enough of the devaluing. She was devaluing our relationship and in turn I was doing it to myself. In my heart I knew what I was doing and it was time to get real with myself. It was time to pursue my dreams. It was time to be alone with me.

❧ Chapter 16 ☙

The Straight World Loves
A Lipstick Lesbian
1995

We walked in, holding our helmets, clear that I had been on the back of his bike, and immediately I could feel the vibe. The girls saw him walk in with me and they were quiet, ignoring, dismissive. I could feel it immediately. I was in straight girl territory and walking into the restaurant could only mean one thing, I was a threat as I may be stealing their boyfriend.

I was told that I looked straight. I took that to mean, I didn't look like a stereotypical queer person because I wore my hair long, which I did mostly since I moved to San Francisco, minus the few years I was trying to fit into the lesbian community that seemed to favor more butch, less femme looks. That didn't work too well for me, being that my hair was wavy and the city fog made it so much more so. So, I suppose my long hair made me a "femme" or a "lipstick lesbian," which were femme women who identified as lesbian or who dated women. And, of course, dark red lipstick was my go-to, giving me color against my dark olive colored skin.

I often was mistaken for being straight. The queer community as a whole didn't like us "lipsticks" much then. I understood why. Our look apes the majority. We get all the privilege of a heteronormative world, but queer when we want to be. How convenient. As a brown person I felt I needed all the help I could get. I always felt long hair looked better on me anyway.

That day, I was with my friend from class. Tall, dark, Alec wore black jeans and leather jackets and rode a motorcycle. Alec definitely had a crush on me. He told me so. And, apparently all the straight girls were into him.

He worked in North Beach, the Italian part of town, as a waiter at a fancy restaurant. He would ride his bike to class, and many nights our little clique from my psychology class and cohort which consisted of Lani, the butch lesbian with the mohawk, Lavender the token straight white girl who slept with black men, Mattie, another musician, psychology major, lesbian who I was close with, Alec, the black leather wearing, motorcycle riding, token straight boy, and myself, the Indian lipstick lesbian, would hang out meeting for drinks in the Mission District after class. This started to become a thing, and eventually a thing I would miss.

I felt accepted by this crowd. In San Francisco, if you weren't dating women, there was something wrong with you.

This night we were hanging out and we needed to stop by his restaurant. The rest of the group had gone ahead to the bar. While riding on the back of Alec's motorcycle, I agreed to first stop at his restaurant.

The tension started the minute those girls laid their eyes on me. At first, they saw Alec walk in the door and big smiles appeared on their faces. They were enamored by Alec and his presence. Then I walked in behind him, helmet in hand, and their smiles faded as quickly as ice cream melts in the summer sun. I just stood there, awkward, wanting to leave. At that moment, Alec stopped talking and turned to me. He must've felt the tension. He introduced me by saying, "Hey everyone, this is Mou." I started to smile and say hello, but before I could finish Alec blurted out, "She's a lesbian."

I was stunned. I had been outed just like that, right then and there, by a straight man, no less. A man I thought was my friend. Immediately, all of my trauma about coming out came flooding back to me. Coming out can be traumatic. For every person who accepts you with open arms, there are 5 more who will shut their door on you. I often remind my clients that coming out never ends, and every time you must come out again, you may get retraumatized again.

But that day, all of a sudden the energy in the room shifted. Immediately the tension was lifted, and a lightness filled the room. The dour female waitresses all immediately perked up and were excited and eager to meet me. They inched closer to me, all smiles and hugs. "Hi, so nice to meet you." Their hands reached forward. "I feel like I should hug you." The red head, who appeared to be the leader of the cold and aloof waitresses, who turns out had dated Alec and held a torch for him, reached out her hand towards me and said, "Here, do you need a light?"

I'd forgotten I was holding a cigarette.

Two things that make a long-haired, straight-looking girl cool in the 1990's San Francisco was her cigarette, her lipstick and her lesbianism. I had officially arrived. Again.

But that was it. I was some sort of torch song, or gateway to the lesbian world, for some straight women that is. But most importantly I was not a threat. I wasn't going to steal their man and even more exciting I might even be attracted to them.

For straight men, I was a safe place to explore their kinks, their fantasies. I wasn't going to shame them. This contrasted with the lesbian world, in which I wasn't so popular.

❧ Chapter 17 ☙

Stocks and Blondes
A Story About Gentle Women
1995

Through Natalia's urging I found myself in a completely strange and unknown world. A world of women who appealed to the male gaze, for the sake of money but slept in the beds of women who donned facial hair, rode motorcycles, played in bands, and wrote poetry. This was the underbelly of San Francisco in the 1990's, the Demi – monde.

And I was learning it was a huge subculture that fed into the more surface queer culture, a weaving of dark alleys under surface streets, water dripping in subway lines after the city had gone to sleep. Lipstick lesbians who now looked like pinup girls in high heeled boots, faux furs and fishnet stockings with their lovers: the leather daddies, drag kings and bearded ladies.

I hadn't gone to too many strip clubs at this point. At my undergraduate program at San Francisco State the biggest class on campus was *Variations in Human Sexuality*, a class on everything BUT heterosexuality. We often had different presenters speak on all the varied subcultures of human sexuality, all of which lived out, open and unabashedly in San Francisco. I remember the day that a slew of strippers and burlesque dancers came and performed in the big auditorium that the class took place in. All of them were students at San Francisco State. It was then that I learned that this was the way many women were making money while studying, paying their way through college, on their way to other careers.

Natalia was an exotic dancer, a stripper. She traveled the world dancing at high end exotic dance clubs and Gentlemen's clubs making lots of money. That's all I knew of. Back then I didn't realize that some of these girls were doing a lot more for a lot more money.

Natalia was visiting San Francisco. She was staying with my latest girlfriend, Barstow, who was also enamored by Natalia. I could smell Natalia's fragrance on my girlfriend's pillow when I would go visit. It was no secret. They slept in the same bed. My girlfriend lived in a small two bedroom with her roommate. Where else would Natalia be sleeping? Besides, Barstow and I were not monogamous.

I was jealous of the adoration more than I was worried that my girlfriend cheated. The adoration was blatant and felt like it was being flanked in my face. For the most part I felt secure in that relationship. My girlfriend had told me many times that she thought I was a catch.

What did make me feel more uncomfortable was Natalia's self-righteous femininity. It felt very similar to the straight girl energy I'd often experienced; judgmental, competitive, spiteful maybe and definitely catty. She didn't hide that she looked down on me. She was better than me. Smarter, prettier, and richer.

Well, she was probably richer. I mean even though I had my degree, I was making close to no money in a social services agency job.

Barstow was busy one night with a gig, and so she encouraged me to go out with Natalia alone.

"I can't join you guys tonight, but you should go. Go out with Natalia."

I didn't want to go without my girlfriend. I had nothing in common with Natalia and didn't feel like she really liked me.

"Yes, come with me," Natalia piped in. She was around often these days.

Sure, why not. Natalia invited me after all. It always feels good to be invited.

And I wanted to play it cool in front of Barstow. I didn't want to let on that Natalia had affected me in any way. Besides, I didn't have my old friend group anymore, so I was happy to have something to do.

That night Natalia took me to the Elbo Room on Valencia Street in the Mission.

I remember what I wore. I was in my new phase of branching out of wearing Doc Martens, leather jackets, flannel shirts, and baggy Levi jeans to wearing more feminine attire. Slightly more feminine boots, still with a chunk but now also with a heel, tight black jeans, and a red button-up blouse. I was wearing my hair curly and long and pinned up on the sides.

For someone who didn't live in town, Natalia knew a lot of people. Elbo Room was clearly her stomping grounds. She was sexy and she knew it, and she flitted around the room saying hi to people who she knew. She would introduce me every now and again as Mou and then go back to her business.

I had been to the Elbo Room before, many times, but tonight I was feeling out of my element. And, yes, it was a predominantly straight place with a lot of diverse music. Tonight, I was an outsider. My current girlfriend wasn't from the same lesbian crowd that I had been used to hanging out with for the past five years. She was part of a new crowd, a more rock'n'roll crowd that mingled amongst men. I was venturing into newer pastures and redefining myself as well. Also, a lot of these people are older than me. I was practically a baby at 23.

But of course, I was old enough to drink. And drink I did. It helped me, of course, look cool and stave off my anxiety. And I drank to the point of getting sick outside of the club. I can't remember much. I do remember I was outside getting sick sitting on the pavement with Natalia by my side. Natalia was telling me that I didn't love myself.

In her oh so sweet and soothing voice, she cooed, "You really need to learn to love yourself." It was more condescending than caring. Even in my stupor I was eye-rolling.

Here she was, sleeping in my girlfriend's bed, riding around the city on my bicycle that my girlfriend convinced me to lend her. Let's be real, that was where my antennae perked up. My girlfriend was giving this girl special attention. But what was so special about Natalia?

Despite feelings of inadequacy coupled with annoyance around Natalia, and my girlfriend, I spent time with them.

And that's how I ended up at Stocks and Blondes.

Stocks and Blondes was a Gentleman's club in San Francisco. Unlike the Lusty Lady which was female owned, and at the forefront of an ongoing movement that was going on at the time of sex workers rallying to unionize, an uprising of women taking their power back not just through sex work but through fighting the labor laws as well, Stocks and Blondes was very male.

Natalia thought I should be embracing my femininity and making money while doing it.

"You're pretty. You should come down and at least check it out."

Okay, why not?

I walked into the club and immediately Natalia introduced me to Maurice. Maurice handled booking all the girls and wanted to know what kind of experience I had.

"What are you drinking?" he asked.

"Vodka gimlet," I told him, even though it had made me so sick just a few nights ago!

He told me to take a seat and check it out and let him know if I wanted a shot; he would give me a shot to go up there and show them what I had.

"Oh, I'm just here to check it out tonight," I reassured him.

I didn't think I was ready to dance!

As I sat at the bar, it was Natalia's turn to go up on the stage. I watched as Natalia who was wearing these 7-inch platform see-through high heels walk up to the stage and started twirling on the pole. I had no experience wearing high heels, let alone dancing on a stripper pole. I was way out of my element. Natalia on the other hand was owning the stage. And, what a workout. No wonder Natalia felt so empowered.

As I was sitting there, one of Natalia's friends, Cinnamon, came and started chatting with me. Cinnamon had just flown in from Maui where she was also dancing. She did the same thing that Natalia did. She would stay in one city for a few weeks, make some money dancing and then move on to the next city. She was living the glamorous life, and she looked it.

Cinnamon was beautiful with her dark brown skin and curly hair, and she was authentically nice. No catty vibes. She was just friendly, and we made small talk.

But these girls were more feminine than I ever could be or even wanted to be. I was sure of it now.

I hung around for probably 30 minutes. I finished my drink and since Natalia was still dancing, I said my goodbyes to Cinnamon, I thanked Maurice for the drink, and I left.

As I walked home in the dark, up Market Street, I was relieved to be out of there. I was not just out of my element, but it was a world I couldn't belong to, no matter how empowered these women were. I couldn't dance or show up for the male gaze like that ever. My feminism didn't involve showing up for men, not even for money. I was clearer than ever about who I was and what I wanted.

A couple years later, I became friends with a gal who worked with me at the agency by day but did camming by night (yes, camming existed in 1996). We hung out a few times before she tried to get me to also do camming.

"This is on camera," she assured me. "You could somewhat hide your identity."

I was struggling for money. So, I entertained the idea. For a split second.

I had always hated the male gaze. Could I use it to make money?

In the end I never did.

I support all choices that women of all colors, body shapes, and genitalia make. Whether they choose sex work or if they get into it because they feel it is their strongest option. I believe that sex work is work, and that erotic labor is valid. I thank these women for these experiences, for giving me the knowledge to make my own informed choices.

Thank you for opening doors for me.

Dead Girls
BY MOUSHUMI GHOSE

I'm back in my city
Where the dead girls sing to me
Cold gray
Long black coat
black boots slipping
Off
Flipping me off
I still hear you

The train rumbles along
This old town
Glittering lights
Unfamiliar faces in these
Old places
This future
I never saw
Oh I know I do
I still hear you

This tube
This tune
I carry you
I still hear you

Dead girls singing
Up to me from
The dark night platform
On these tracks
Way below
They hear me too
They still hear me too

❧ Chapter 18 ❦

The Musical Girls
1996

I was supposed to meet the girls that night after the show, but I had to drive Lucia home first. I told Colette that I would be back in 15 minutes and then we would all go "party."

I knew Colette through Barstow, who I dated briefly. Colette and Barstow were musicians. Barstow had been my rescue when I couldn't take it anymore. Nell had repeatedly broken non-monogamy agreements with me. My heart was in pieces.

Oh, how I loved Barstow and everything she represented. She was also a woman of color, a lesbian, a musician and to my heart's delight, and what we initially bonded over, was that she had just returned from a soul-searching trip to India. In 1995, it was rare for me to meet anyone who had traveled to India. I had been traveling to India myself back and forth since I was a little child and often felt so disjointed, disconnected, and lost when I would return. The night I met Barstow I too had recently returned from India. I immediately felt a connection.

Barstow and I sat at the bar that night and talked for hours it seemed. I told her how my best friend and I hit the road for a month, traveling all over India and South East Asia. And, how it had been life changing for me. This had been a profound trip because it was the first time in my life I was able to share my experience with an American peer. None of my white peers understood what it meant to be a daughter of immigrants from India.

Barstow nodded yes. I felt so seen, for the first time in a long time.

I continued, "It was legendary to see India through Lynda's eyes. I had seen this so many times through my parent's eyes, poverty, struggle, dirt, and grime, seeing this through Lynda's eyes, made my love for India and travel to foreign lands grow into a lifelong passion." Barstow could relate to this.

We shared our stories. So many similarities. From sunrises at the Taj Mahal to the quaint village of Bhaktapur in Kathmandu at the foot of the Himalayas, to swimming at dusk on a rooftop in Bangkok, and getting sick with the runs in Jaipur. I even told Barstow of how my heart had shattered. How I shared everything so openly with Lynda, my "best girlfriend," about my troublesome open relationship with Nell. I said, "But I'm so into her."

"Aww man," Barstow exclaimed.

That night I met Barstow, I was still devastated from my best friend's betrayal, and still barely hanging on with Nell. My heart was raw. I was underwater.

Sitting there with Barstow, I felt she would understand. After all, we weren't actually on a date, anyway. We'd just met.

Nell and I had been adhering to our "one fuck rule." In other words, we were still dating. We could sleep with one person without telling each other. But after the second time, we had to spill the beans. "If you sleep with someone a second time, you are going to catch feelings," Nell would say.

I went along with Nell's rules. In theory, they made a lot of sense to me. But I was hurting inside. She was sleeping with our friends, her roommates, straight women, gay women, ex-girlfriends, you name it. (I wish I had known I could negotiate the terms of our relationship. She might have respected me more had I spoken up.)

To top it off, I confided all of my heartache to Lynda during our trip. Lynda listened to me while I talked about this. I was so madly in love with Nell and was hurting. Lynda didn't say anything and just listened.

And upon returning from our trip, one of the first things I did was see Nell. She had missed me and was excited to see me. I was ecstatic to see her. As we lay there, having just made love, I began to tell her all about my trip.

Lynda and I had a great time, and she met my family.

"Oh my god, she had such culture shock when we first arrived in India."

I was elated as I relayed the story to her. I finally was doing something important that I could brag about, that was making me feel better. I felt like I was finally finding myself.

Nell interrupted me and said, "Um, Lynda is not your friend."

"What do you mean? Lynda is my best friend. We are so close. We would do anything for each other."

"Nope. She wouldn't. She is not your best friend."

I couldn't understand what she was saying. Why would she…

She started talking, "Before you left for India, Lynda and I…" and then it hit me. Lynda and Nell had hooked up.

I had never in a million years suspected that the "don't ask, don't tell" aspect of our relationship would extend to best friends. I was devastated to find out that it did in fact include my very so-called best friend. Nell was under no obligation to disclose anything to me per the "agreement" we had. But my best friend keeping it from me felt completely unethical and wrong. Wasn't there some sort of best friend code? Apparently not. I'd have to negotiate for that, too!

We were supposed to have a date at 7 PM, but by 9 PM she hadn't called or shown up and I was beside myself. She was over two hours late when I finally got the call.

"Sorry I missed our date. Emma stopped by and wanted to try to work things out."

Emma was Nell's ex.

Just one week prior, Nell had given me the dolphin ring to solidify our commitment. We were going to try monogamy. All Nell's idea. I just went along with it. Easy going. Poop.

Then one night, after getting off the phone with Nell, heart crashing in my stomach, I was beside myself. Not knowing what to do, I called up the butchest dyke friend I had, Mohawk wearing Estella who picked me up in her Suzuki Samurai jeep and sped us over to the Transmission lounge bar south of Market, and then I met Barstow.

I wish this had a happily ever after ending. But when I started seeing Barstow, I broke not just the "one fuck rule" I also threw Nell's plans for a "commitment" out the window, without nary a discussion. Things got messy after that. You see I had enough of going along with it and I just woke up one day and I flipped. It's funny how the body will just tell you. I still loved Nell, but it was time to take back the reins.

But Barstow and I had fun. We were an attractive multiracial non-white couple, she was more masculine with her dreads, and me a femme lipstick lesbian. We flaunted ourselves at the Folsom Street Fair, then the Castro Street Fair that year and imagined a long life together. She introduced me to her friends. A completely new lesbian friend circle full of musicians and social justice academics, but the key here is imagined because a few months into it the cracks would appear in our shiny veneer.

On a Sunday afternoon, after she had been busy for several days, she showed up at my doorstep.

"Hey, I wanted to tell you that Natalia and I haven't slept together yet, but it might happen. I just wanted to be honest with you in case something does happen." (Yes, Natalia the stripper had been staying with Barstow. Don't worry, I knew about it, and I had to trust Barstow.)

My heart broke once again. Barstow was so sweet and respectful to give me this information. It was honest. However, that doesn't mean it didn't hurt.

I took a deep breath, kept my composure, smiled at her and said, "Thank you for letting me know. I had a feeling." And then, it just came tumbling out of my mouth. I didn't want her to see me sad, weak, so I took the upper hand.

I said, "We should take a break, I think it's a good time to take a break."

She acted surprised. "You want to take a break?"

"Yea, I think we should. Take some time and space so we can both figure out what we want."

"Really? Okay. Sure. That sounds like a good idea." And with tears in her eyes, she agreed. I don't think she expected me to be so strong about it. So decisive. I even surprised myself. Initially, I had wanted to say, "No problem, we will be fine, enjoy yourself," but somehow saying it like that made me feel like a pushover, revisiting my life with Nell all over again. I had agreed to the rules with Nell, I didn't try to negotiate or set any parameters of my own, I just went along with something that was hurting me time and time again. I wasn't going to let that happen again. So, I said goodbye to Barstow, even though my heart was crashing to the floor.

I never saw Barstow around in San Francisco much after that as she was off on tour. I guess breaking up had freed her to pursue her truth! And then I bumped into Colette several months later at a concert at Slim's. Throwing Muses had since broken up, but I was excited to see their female front person and songwriter up front and personal. It was a good show. At the time I was barely beginning my own songwriting journey.

After exchanging niceties and introducing me to her cool musician friends, Colette said, "Come with us. We're gonna party."

"I will. Wait here for me, I'll be back in 15 minutes." I desperately wanted to hang out with them. I was there with Lucia, and ever since Barstow and I had split up, I had been out of the lesbian scene completely. Lucia was straight. Which in and of itself was fine, but she was an introvert. She didn't drink. She didn't socialize much. She definitely didn't party, at least not those days. And, I had been ostracized from the queer world because I was dating men.

I was also scared because I knew what the San Francisco punk band scene was all about.

Heroin.

And it was kind of glamorous to me. But I was also scared to try it. In recent years, I heard of quite a few overdoses of friends, friends of friends and acquaintances. And I'd heard it was making its rounds through the music scene in San Francisco as well. I really wanted more access to music, art and creativity. I was stuck in academia. Going to party with them could open doors. And I knew if I went to party with them, it would be on the table. I might try it. But not much. Or not at all. But who knows? What I did know, I wanted to hang out with more musicians. I kept my eyes on the prize.

I made it back to the club after driving Lucia home. I had actually grown quite tired by then. I was also not the type to flake. Dutiful, responsible me. Always pleasing (read: trauma response?). I didn't want her to be waiting. I didn't want that to be the story. So, I showed up. I looked around, and the club was empty by then. No one was there. Just a few stragglers, and Colette and her friends were nowhere in sight. I didn't linger too long. It was dark. I hurriedly got in the car and drove home.

As I drove home it occurred to me that this scene was not for me. As much as I wanted to meet more cool, rock'n'roll femme and queer musicians, I just knew I could not and should not go down that dark road.

I was tired. At 23 I had finished school, gotten my first full-time adult job, was trying to create my art, and had my heart broken by so many women, both lovers and friends alike. I thought non-monogamy would be easier, but that turned out to be just as hard. Again, I began to wonder where my people were at.

Velveteen
BY MOUSHUMI GHOSE

Summer and spring
I don't know where I've been
I don't know who I am
What I'm doing
What's this
In between

Velveteen like silk pants
Rubber plants
Pink slacks

Velveteen jacket on your lapel
Shoulder holster
You know so well

I'm tired
So tired
Laborious labor
Lifeguard
Afraid

‰ Chapter 19 ‰

Distress and Disorientation
1997

Distress and disorientation can happen in one's youth and may result from conflicting tensions and ambiguity about yourself and your role in society as a whole.

We live in a world where everyone tries to keep up with the Joneses. As a non-white girl I wanted to fit in from the age of 5, which was around the time I started to notice that I did not look like everyone else. I compared myself to the girls around me, going as far back as I can remember.

My story is that being bisexual and fluid granted me a lot of freedoms. It opened my eyes to the types of people who I related to.

Embracing my sexual fluidity was the key to my liberation. I was able to stop comparing myself to others, started living my best life, and began healing my trauma. But it was a long road ahead. I had more learning and exploration to do.

After dating only women for several years, I had had enough. I was making my way through girlfriends faster than I was going through my shoes. I felt it in my bones. I was getting stagnant, and I needed change. Even attending the annual dyke march at PRIDE was boring. I needed something else, and fast. So, with the blink of an eye, I started flirting with and dating men. Rooted in toxic masculinity, this was a difficult move for a feminist queer woman like me, but I thought I needed to be true to my intrinsic sexual and human nature.

I used to separate the personal from the political. Dating women was very much political for me. As a feminist, heteronormativity and traditional male and female roles felt oppressive to me, and then discovering at 16 a world where I was not only attracted to women, but could also be with them, changed my life. But the truth is, I had also always been attracted to men.

During my years with women, this plagued me a bit. I loved the lesbian community and everything it stood for. The lesbian community of San Francisco was pretty militant. It had no time for the patriarchy, heteronormativity. It was kinky, playful and extremely fluid, but it was not without its limitations. If you were a woman, you could be a butch, a baby dyke, a femme, but there was no room for bisexuality in that world. And, suddenly, the stakes felt like they were getting higher. The deeper I got involved in the lesbian community, it felt the further I would drift away into a darkness of girls who used knives during sexy play, hard drugs, and I didn't know what else. And I was a little too vanilla for that.

Instead, after I began dating men, I quickly drifted away from the lesbian community.

"I'm dating a guy now," led to distraught faces and reactions like, "Oh, so you're bisexual?"

"Yea, yea, I guess I am." Insert sad face here. I was a traitor, and I hated myself for it.

***NOTE: This was the 1990's. We didn't have terms like Pansexual, Fluid, or the LGBTQIA umbrella to explain our identity. Queer was still a term used to describe mostly gay and lesbian only. The gay and lesbian communities were also synonymous with the Kink communities back then as well.

Then, at best their attention would wane, they would slowly lose interest, their eyes would no longer sparkle, their smiles would dwindle or become fake. Worse was that they would huff loudly, "Ugh," or express disdain out loud, like, "Ewwww, that's so gross," and/or blatantly turnaround and walk away and start talking to someone else. Cue: abandonment trauma. My fuck-a-bility was now gone.

Women who identify as Bi. Yes, they ape the majority, while perpetuating the patriarchy, toxic masculinity, heteronormativity. I understood it all too well.

One thing led to another, and very quickly I found myself living with a man. I guess I was in love, for the force was strong enough to pull me away from my lesbian identity. Sure, I was calling myself bisexual, and had been for the better part of that decade, when not referring to myself as a lesbian or a dyke, but in my heart, I knew that bisexuality was not a thing most people understood or wanted to acknowledge.

I was alienated. I could no longer go to The Café and mingle openly. At some point my relationship status would come up, and, well, I was living with a man.

I had a few girlfriends left who I would mingle with outside of the bars. It was slim pickings. I didn't enjoy the heteronormative world of family BBQs.

What happened to the days when we all hung out together, like in high school when everyone identified as bisexual and anything went? There had to be something different.

Lonely and sad, I drifted through my days. I'd met some girls through work, straight girls who didn't clique around with a straight girl crew, and so on the weekends I would spend my time with them, when I wasn't with my boyfriend. I also spent my days alone, not sure where I belonged nor what to do with myself.

I had become my own worst nightmare. Straight poop.

One sunny summer day, I took the afternoon off work and I decided to do a little clothes shopping. I headed up to Market Street to my favorite thrift store at the time, Crossroads.

I was sifting through the racks and racks of clothing. I still needed to look stylish, right?

"Mou, is that you?" I looked up and a petite girl with curly strawberry blonde hair was looking back at me. It took me a minute to register who it was. It was Kourtney. Kourtney had dated Lea for a while a few years ago. She must not have gotten the memo yet that I was dating men.

"Oh, hey, Kourtney," I said cautiously. I knew how this was going to end, once she found out I was dating a man.

"How are you? What's going on?"

"Oh, nothing much, just buying some new clothes." Obvious and bored.

We engaged in small talk about how stylish she thought I was, cue: the blushing, and mused about how so much had changed since we last saw one another.

"Was it two years ago?"

"Yes, since Lea and I broke up."

I knew a lot had changed for me, but had no idea what she was referring to. I guess you could say my interest was piqued. Though, admittedly, lesbian drama had lost its spark and bordered on tedium these days.

"You know, I am dating a man now," I blurted out.

I often felt the need to come clean about dating men with most of my lesbian friends. It was almost like I needed to remind them that there was a world outside of the lesbian community. San Francisco had gotten small.

Kourtney smiled and continued casually surfing through the racks of used clothing. "We need to hang out, Mou." She held up a top. "This one would look cute on you!" It was way too small, but I appreciated the style.

"Hey, what are you doing right now? I mean, after you finish here. Wanna go grab a coffee at Du Nord?" she asked. Du Nord was right up the block. A coffee house that also served alcohol right in the heart of the gay part of town, one block away from Castro Street.

Surprised that she was serious about hanging out, but also thrilled to have something to do that afternoon, I replied, "Yea, sure."

What did I have to lose? I guess I'd listen if she wanted to share news of her newest lady dalliances, and I could have a new friend to hang out with. Kourtney didn't seem to mind I was dating a man.

That afternoon was the start of a new friendship. Thanks to Kourtney, I felt found again. We chatted at Du Nord for hours over Irish coffee and beignets.

That day over coffee, Kourtney told me she was also bisexual. She had been dating a man.

"You should come out with us this Friday. We're going to have dinner."

Oh cool. Sure, I'd go hang out with some bi girls. Why not?

But it wasn't dinner after all. In fact, we never even made it to the restaurant.

Kourtney was dating one man, but she was sleeping with many men... at the sex clubs of San Francisco. She would go to the clubs, strap on a dildo and fuck gay men in the ass. She was also dating women. Many of these women were also bisexual.

Kourtney had a large friend circle, too. Straight women, bi women, bi men and gay men.

And there were drugs. Lots of drugs. But it was San Francisco. It was the 1990's. I didn't really think much of it. I had already been there and done that anyway.

Yes, a lot had changed. Our lesbian days when she was dating Lea, seemed oh so very tame compared to this.

That night, about 10 more people gathered at Kourtney's place "to go to dinner," but we missed our 9 PM reservation, and it was well past 1 AM when we made it to the after-hours sex club. Drugs will make you lose track of all time. But what a fun night for the books. I needed this after my year of distress and disorientation. I needed this reset.

My world had opened up again. This was what I had been looking for. Wasn't it? But, I could feel the uncertainty. The anxiety. The unsustainability. The sex clubs were great fun. But combined with the endless drugs, it all seemed like part of a dark underworld where one could get lost and never return from. And many did. My steady head would never allow me to drift too far from the shore. I feared this friend group would only be temporary.

I was one foot in, one foot out. I stayed an outsider, although I would've welcomed open arms. I jumped in when and where I could, when Kourtney would invite me, but I didn't always get an invite. I took the drugs, for a day, an afternoon, an evening, once or twice a month, before finding my way back home to my boyfriend on Sunday night to prepare for the week ahead, while many of the others partied on into the work week, and who knows when they came up for air, if ever.

Still, I felt that, in that year of loss and isolation, this was better than hanging out with the straights. Certainly, it was better than being alone, and I had found an opening.

This was life in my queer utopia, San Francisco in the 1990's. A subculture that could not legally marry, did not have any rights, lived underground on the fringes of society. No rights also meant in most cases support was missing from biological families too, and a general disconnect from the world at large. The gay community of the 1990's survived because of friends, and what is often referred to as "chosen family." These friends created bonds and provided mutual support and love to each other. This was Kourtney and her friends' chosen family. I had lost much of my chosen family when I started dating men.

I still look back on my life that year. Bumping into Kourtney that day was a great reminder that what you want, what you need is out there. Trust the process. Trust in yourself. Get out in the world and live.

It's not always going to be perfect. It will sometimes be hard. But you keep going.

Your people are out there.

The Girl for the Revolution
BY MOUSHUMI GHOSE

There's a girl
So deep
There's a girl
She goes
She suffers
She cries
She's got the weight of the world
But she goes
And where she goes
I wanna go
I wanna follow

She leads the world
In her quiet sorrow
Deafening anger
Scary scowl
But she knows
Therefore she goes

And when the revolution comes
I wanna go
For she will lead us all out of
This mess

Chapter 20

The Tears of Sexually Liberated Women: An Essay Spanning 35 Years 1985-2021

2021

She called me in tears. Bawling her eyes out. She did not understand what she did wrong. She loved him so much. She was devastated.

My heart broke as I listened to her cry. She was this strong woman who did not take shit. She ran her own business. She put herself out there. Sure, she often got punched (literally and figuratively) and she would get right back up. This was the first time I heard her balling like this. She loved him so much. She would do anything to get him back. Including quitting her job.

This client was an adult performer and a sex worker. As many of my clients are. In fact, in my work as a therapist, many of my clients live on the fringe sexually, relationally, non-normative, outside the box, outside of what is considered normal, acceptable, upstanding and so on. My job and mission has been to help those of us who do live on the fringe, find a voice to be able to live more authentically. The hardest job in the world, really, I am constantly swimming upstream. I enjoyed the work for a long time. I always knew I was helping people, supporting people on their most difficult journey, life. But how could I help them find authentic voices when I was burnt out from fighting the fight? I no longer could.

That day, despite my burnout, and likely because of it, I broke down in tears after I got off the phone with my client. I have been fighting this fight for a long time and this client was not easy. You see, trauma begets trauma. You've heard the saying, "Hurt people hurt people," right? This was the same client who just a year ago had yelled at me, fought with me, distrusted me in the beginning and tried to fire me, several times.

At times, I hated working with her. And, as a therapist, I knew better. I knew her anger was not about me. I knew there were deeper things at play. I knew that my behavior, my language, my words had struck a nerve, or as we say in therapist speak, had triggered her, and she was responding from her trauma by reacting, automatically, and without thinking. This trauma I have been witnessing and fighting all my life.

Over that last year and half, I had gotten to know this client. She was trying hard to make money, to be a respectable adult, and to live a fulfilling life. In prior years she had gotten sober, she had worked to stop many of her blatant self-defeating behaviors, but of course despite being sober, many of the behaviors were still showing up, as they often do. Closure is not a thing that really exists. Things come back up in our lives. We just get better at recognizing their effects and managing them.

As a sex positive psychotherapist, I am one of few therapists who could support her in her treatment and not make therapy all about her work. Unfortunately, her partner did make their relationship all about her work.

Our society still does not accept sex work as a professional form of work. And what often starts out as a well-meaning relationship, eventually the men cannot handle her professions. She had seen this all too often. So had I. Still, she was blaming herself. *Where did she go wrong?*

This was not the first time I would experience this phone call. You see, this is a call that many women will make.

Sexual freedom for women is never free. It comes at a cost. Men are allowed to sow their oats. Women do it too but beware as it may come to bite you in the ass.

1985

I was barely 13, not sure what I would even do with boys. We met the boys by hanging around in the downtown area of our small suburb. Then my good friend, also 13 and "boy crazy" (one who would give anything for the attention of the boys) began actually hooking up with one of the boys, to my surprise, while I waited in the living room watching TV with one of the other boys. No one made a move on me. I was not the one that boys wanted to hook up with. So, I got the job of a friend. This was the norm in those early years.

Once, I walked by the bedroom where my friend was hooking up with one of the hot boys from downtown. I heard him say, "Stroke it, faster, harder." What? My 13-year-old ears were mortified, disgusted, and felt so scared for my friend. Men and boys seemed to have the upper hand. I wanted action, however in reality I just wanted to be liked, but I knew then there was no way in hell I was going to be subservient for it. I didn't want that kind of awkward sexual action. I was relieved in that moment that it was not me. Did I mention I was 13? Penises still grossed me out.

Later, I got the phone call.

"I haven't gotten my period."

"He hasn't called me back. Will you call him and pretend…?"

"Pretend what?"

Some kind of manipulation to get a 14-year-old boy, who is still a child and too young, and who probably was not yet taught how to treat a young woman, to call her back. If only she could get his attention.

The next day we were going downtown again. This time another friend joined us. She hooked up with his brother.

"How was it?" I asked.

"When he was on top of me, a drop of sweat fell on me."

"Sounds romantic."

"It was gross," she said dryly, with a hint of disgust in her voice.

Um. What is the point of that? I thought to myself. What did these girls want? And, also a hint of why does no guy want me?

Several weeks later, she is sobbing on the phone.

"I just took a pregnancy test. I need to get an abortion. How am I going to pay for it?"

At the time, early 1980's, an abortion at Planned Parenthood cost $267, a lot of money for our teenage selves. And of course, she couldn't tell her parents.

I met her at her house after school the day of the abortion. She didn't talk much as it was, and I could tell from her demeanor that she definitely wasn't in the mood today. We took the bus downtown in silence, so she could get it "taken care of." I waited in the lobby until it was done. Finally, an hour later, maybe two, she came out and said, "Let's go."

We took the bus back to her house, and then I took the bus back to my house. I didn't get home until 9 PM, and my mother was worried.

"Where were you?"

"Studying at Steph's."

A few months later Steph was nowhere to be seen. She'd found a new crowd to hang with and she was absent from school a great deal. She had met a seductively attractive blonde girl, who was older, and she would attract even hotter, more influential boys. They were dating musicians, and these boys were much older than us. She bleached her dark hair blonde and told me with great pride that she was getting more catcalls than ever walking down the street. She felt good about this. She was going back for more. It would likely never end. She would kill for the attention from the boys. Of course, I was unable to get what she was getting. I wasn't blonde and while she spoke I felt a tinge of envy. "Wow, to be beautiful and desired," but it was fleeting, as well as feeling out of reach, and I was okay with that because, deep down, I knew the cost was too steep.

I consoled my friends when guys broke up with them and ghosted them. I accompanied them when they needed to go to planned parenthood to get abortions. I got to observe firsthand much larger elements at play. Boys barely had to show up. Get chased. Get off. Disappear. Pursue their dreams of skateboarding, being a musician, howling in the night. Girls were left holding the bag.

I felt sad for these girls, who did not know their worth. On the other hand, I wanted excitement and fun too. The question however, wasn't whether I would give up all my feminism if they showered me with their attention. The question was: how do I get around this toxic masculinity and learn to play as an equal? These girls gotta play, but there was no equality in this play. I knew there had to be another way.

Almost a decade later I would date men, but it would be after a debaucherous decade of sexual liberation in the queer world. I had found equality in the queer world, and so I thought I was so different from these girls. I thought I was removed from the dangers of the heteronormative world. I was queer after all.

He had loved that I had only had relationships with women. He said I was a breath of fresh air from the heterosexual women he'd encountered who were, "Dick-oriented." Of course, what this really meant was his ego got to stay intact because I wasn't messing around with other boys which also made me safe. This was a good thing for him. But I fell for it. Hook, line and sinker.

What he hadn't accounted for, was that I was not "dick oriented" which translates to I was not on board for the entitlement men have towards sex, pleasure, and female bodies. What he initially loved about me, I was gay, later became the problem.

Maybe he thought he could fuck the lesbian out of me, train me. Maybe he thought, because of my long hair, "She is not really a lesbian." But when the sex faltered, I heard this: "I don't know if you're cheating on me with Tom, Dick, Harry or Mary." Yet, I wasn't cheating on him.

The relationship felt so imbalanced. At times it felt like he wanted me to stay at home and wait for him, while he went out and had all the fun. Double standards. Different rules for women than what is expected of men. And, toxic masculinity. Boys and girls being raised with the belief that women are here to serve, be afraid, stay indoors, and second class citizens, and that a woman who describes herself as a lesbian would ultimately want to be with a man. That the sex is all about the men, too.

That relationship was the death of me. I can see it so clearly now as hindsight is 20/20. I had been dating women for the last decade and was ready for the next phase in my sexual evolution. I was ready to have sex with men, but I was nowhere near prepared for what it means to date men as a woman. I did not subscribe to the rules of heterosexuality, heteronormativity. I was ill-equipped for the straight world. From the outside I looked like a sexually liberated woman. But what does that mean? It meant simply, I slept with women *and* men.

Many men I talk to, mostly my white male clients, abhor the idea of toxic masculinity, but they don't recognize that it has hurt them too. Toxic masculinity is what makes them fearful of other men taking their women, fearful of humiliation by another man, jealousy. One of my clients called it toxic femininity. He is correct. Toxic femininity comes out of toxic masculinity. Women being catty with each other, and not having each other's backs comes from toxic masculinity. Men are in power in a patriarchal society. Men make the rules. Maybe not the specific men who show up in my therapy office, or the average Joe walking down the street. They may not feel that they have any say in the rules of sexuality, but they do. Sex in our heteronormative world is geared towards them, geared towards men.

In recent years, I have become more and more aware of this privilege, the toxic gender roles and deeply rooted misogyny that underlies so much of our rules when it comes to sex and relationships. As the industry of mental health slowly shifts towards social justice, our work needs to do this, and gets to do this too. And yet, this is where the rubber meets the road. Learning about toxic masculinity has made my job at least that much harder. Because not all men are ready to hear this.

I had been fighting for a cause that I did not have words for. Toxic Masculinity. Heteronormativity. The Patriarchy. I could encourage people to embrace their sexual fluidity, but how was I going to teach our men, and women, about the greater oppressive system at large?

I was not prepared to be in a relationship with a man. Here I was, a queer, sexually liberated woman who had had threesomes, and foursomes and orgies with lots of men and women, and yet I did not know how to play the rules of the hetero club. At the ripe old age of 23, I had lived a full life, and yet somehow, I had missed out on heterosexuality 101. Women and men bowing to the patriarchy.

My politics were not in alignment with what my body wanted. My brain and body were out of sync. The problem was I was really enjoying penetrative sex and to reap the benefits I thought I had to embrace heterosexual sex, I thought I had to play the game. I had to learn about male sexuality, in all its misogynistic, toxic masculinity glory - the pride and joy of the patriarchy. But I had to learn. It was inevitable. So, I did. I told myself I was learning how to ape the majority, and I took a deep dive into heteronormative sex.

↯ Chapter 21 ↯

Lovely Lily
1997

She was nice, but the story I was telling everyone at the time was that she had gotten clingy. As though treating someone with compassion and calling someone after you build a rapport and have a connection with was a bad thing. Truth be told, in other circumstances, I would have welcomed her attention.

"It's all about timing," a friend had said to me just a few years back. It was true. Just a few years ago when I had been in an open relationship with a woman, I would have loved to have met this lovely creature, who was doting, stylish, who loved to travel and really had all the qualities I wanted in a girlfriend – or even just a friend. But after a botched stint in non-monogamy when my heart had been broken into pieces by a woman, my fear of abandonment kicked into high-gear, and I found myself in a monogamous relationship with a male partner.

After dating mostly women for eight years, my last two relationships with women being open, I decided it was time to date a man. I was repeating all the old stuff, yet, now I was choosing something different, I thought, so outside of my lane… men.

If you'd asked me then, why, I would say men felt safer, emotionally, at least, but I wouldn't have been able to put the burden I felt into words. But, now I can. Privilege. Men have privilege in our world, as do heterosexual couples. As a bisexual woman, I have the PRIVILEGE to slide in and out of this. Sure, at the time it felt safer, easier, in some ways, than queer, kinky, and open relationships. But there was a cost... my identity.

I had been wading in the deep end of the queer waters for years and was drowning. I was sick and tired of being sick and tired. Anxious. Unable to sleep. I was getting hurt by these women and I wasn't focused. I wasn't focusing on myself nor my art. I needed stability.

It would have taken true grit then to stay with women, be open, and explore my bisexual side with men, while also getting deeper into kink. It could have been transformational. And I suddenly had no interest in it anymore. Or I feared it. I feared being more alone than I already was. I was tired and weary. So, I jumped in with both feet with this guy. Straight to Hetero-Monogamous-ville.

In my defense it was my first stint in exploring heterosexual relationships and I was a little lost, having had only dated women and only living within a very queer, kinky community for eight years. I was in over my head. But I was attracted to him. And back then I hadn't developed a voice to speak up about non-monogamy. I was well versed in speaking up about my bisexuality, but few really understood polyamory then.

And that's when I met Lily.

At 6-foot 1, Lily was tall, had a slight build, with short shiny black hair. She had almond shaped eyes, and her style was Asian inspired, thrift store immaculate with the perfect amounts of leather and silk, and of course motorcycle boots.

She'd grown up in the US, Asia and Hawaii. As a first-generation born to south-Asian immigrant parents myself, I craved this multi-cultural understanding. She was equal parts masculine and feminine, American and Asian, she loved to travel. We talked about traveling to Thailand and Vietnam, and having only recently discovered my love for travel having traveled around southeast Asia and India myself, I felt I'd suddenly met my soulmate. If I believed in such a thing.

The problem was I had just moved in with a boy.

So, what to do? Well as any self-respecting bisexual polyamorous girl would do in the 1990's, I was going to hang out with this lovely creature, and deal with it. Besides, I was going to rule the school my way as I had always done.

Lily and I started spending more time together. She wanted to take me out (not a date) and to meet her after work. I showed up at her work. She was working at a theater on Haight Street. She was wearing a white shirt unbuttoned with a black tie tied loosely around her neck. It wasn't fully her style, but it was still sexy.

"Hi." She beamed. She seemed happy to see me.

"Hey." I smiled back. I was happy to see her.

We spent the evening riding around San Francisco on her motorcycle. We got Thai food at her favorite spot in lower heat then we grabbed dessert at a really cute café in Japantown.

We ended up at her apartment. It was a typical apartment for San Francisco, tucked away in a cute little neighborhood in Hayes Valley. The radiator was humming in her one bedroom apartment making the space toasty.

Lily set about turning on lights and lamps which were covered with Asian scarves and fabrics. There was art on the walls and trinkets everywhere. The house smelled like soap and incense.

"Come here," she said, sitting on her bed. I went and sat down obediently. "Open your mouth."

I did. She placed something on my tongue. We'd earlier spoken about taking LSD or mushrooms together sometime in the near future, to which she had informed me, "I have a little at home."

"Just a little acid," she said now, followed by, "it's not much."

I didn't spit it out nor object. I was such a people pleaser. *I guess we're doing this.*

As we started talking on her bed, I could feel myself sinking into her. I was getting comfortable. I was also getting aroused, and I could feel our closeness building. I was feeling high. I was feeling good. Suddenly, I looked up. I noticed the clock. I pulled away.

"I have to go," I said apologetically.

"You do?" She seemed surprised. "Why?"

"Yea." I knew my live-in boyfriend would be waiting. I'd officially become one of those girls I despised. Straight and secretive. Dishonest. The worst kind of person.

I packed up my stuff, gave her a quick hug and then left in a hurry.

Of course, he was not happy when I got home.

A few weeks prior when Lily and I had first met she called me three times the following day, leaving sweet messages on our answering machine.

I'm so glad to meet you.

I can't wait to share this new restaurant with you.

Hope you are having an amazing day.

But that was three times too many for my boyfriend. He was beyond suspicious.

"Why would you hang out with someone who clearly is into you?"

He was right. I knew what I was doing.

I'm lonely. My heart screamed. *I need friends.* Lots and lots of friends. And I was non-monogamous, but I never told him I still wanted this, needed this. Not to mention, his words told me everything I needed to know.

Tell him.

I just knew it wasn't going to be accepted and I'd lose him. But ever since I had stopped dating women I had lost my entire community. I had one straight girlfriend and we'd been spending a lot of time together. I was in a dark place.

Lily was a breath of fresh air.

But I never said those things aloud. I was ashamed. And I didn't think he would understand anyway.

As he and I fought over the phone calls, he said, "You must like her." My blood felt like it was boiling.

"Well you are always out with your guy friends," I shot back, as though I was doing this in retaliation. I wasn't.

"Yes, but she is a lesbian. She likes you." I couldn't argue with that. I liked her too.

Tell him.

I didn't say a word. I chickened out, and instead I became irrational. "Fine, I will call her right now and tell her to stop calling."

I dialed *69.

"Hello," she answered, "Tower House," she was working at the theater.

"Please don't call here anymore," I blurted, my vision still blurry, heart racing.

"I thought we were going to be friends," she said calmly but concerned.

"Yes, but you are being disrespectful to my relationship."

UGH.

"I'm so sorry. I didn't mean to call you that much. I'm so sorry."

I hung up on her. My heart hurt.

She was heavy handed with the phone calls, but she didn't deserve that.

I called her first thing in the morning from work.

"I'm sorry about yesterday. My boyfriend is jealous and insecure. Call me at work so it doesn't have to be in his face anymore."

That's when the secrecy started.

We talked several times at work and hung out on the down low. Don't ask, don't tell. Out of sight and out of mind. Heteronormative, straight, monogamous poop. That's what I'd become. Until that night high on acid I could've stayed much longer and let the relationship go further. But I chose not to.

After I left her apartment, I never went back. I knew this friendship would never work out as long as I was with my boyfriend. Lily and I lost touch.

Being in that relationship brought out the worst in me, in many ways. Loneliness was big. And, although he was my boyfriend and we lived together, he was no replacement for community. In fact, he spent a lot of time with "the guys." A very toxic heterosexual trope and binary characteristic I was just not familiar with. A huge red flag I chose to ignore. And of course, he was traditional and monogamous.

Eventually, I became reacquainted with some queer, fluid girls from the club scene who were more accepting of my current relationship, and spent time with them. When I would see Lily out at bars, because I still frequented the lesbian bars despite having a boyfriend, the story was, "She got clingy and I had to break it off."

And, when my boyfriend and I finally broke up, which we were destined to do, (I mean the red flags were insane, but that's a whole other story for another time) so many years later, Lily and I reconnected and we have stayed friends. We tried to date again, but I learned she doesn't really believe in non-monogamy, though I think with her as with many people, once people learn to feel secure in non-monogamy, and polyamory, their views on it can change. Also, the labels are activating for a lot of people.

Today, her friendship and loyalty are deep. I would consider her to be a best friend. And years later this is what Lily, who prides herself as a "gold star lesbian" – someone who has never slept with a man, had to say about our time together and her time with other "bi" girls:

"Bisexual girls really fucked with me. We would fool around, and you all would have your fun, but when it came down to it the bi girls always go back to their boyfriends."

I couldn't have summarized it any better.

ᵔᵔ Chapter 22 ᵔᵔ

The Personal Is Political: We Have Work to Do

I stood there in my cream-colored, sequined evening gown as one of my closest friends said, "You have to come. You cannot waste that dress."

Of course, I was going. I was the life of the party. I rarely, if ever, missed out. I started to speak, "Yes…" but my words trailed off as my partner whispered in my ear, "Um, you're not going out tonight. We just got married."

It was then that I knew I had made a mistake.

At 29, I had been bored. I was staring down 30 and I thought my life was slipping away. Was it not time to get married?

Despite all the signs to the contrary, including my own personal beliefs, I ended up in the most heterosexual of relationships, with the most heterosexual guy.

My politics were betraying my body and I was driven by a strange desire. One year turned into 3 years, which turned into let's move to Los Angeles, where I finally made friends, and for the first time in a long time, my sexual preference wasn't a controversy.

"Oh, you used to date women?"

"Cool."

And marrying a guy didn't seem all that bad, although I always knew it wasn't my whole story. And, once in LA, I openly shared my bisexual past. Yes, that's how it was often referred to, as something I had done "in the past."

But, I wore it like a badge of honor. I used to date women. I am still bisexual.

I wouldn't end up going to the party that night. It was a rave on a boat, and all my queer San Francisco friends were going.

"No, I won't be making it tonight."

I had made a choice and I was going to honor it, although my heart sank. I was under the impression that things would stay the same after getting married. We would continue to live our carefree, independent lives, parties and all.

I kept repeating, "Nothing is going to change." Although I think he gave me hints to the contrary.

But, he might have asked me, "Do you really want to be married?" or warned me, "Things are going to be different once we are married."

But, I wasn't listening.

"Of course I want to be married."

And, I stayed in the relationship for another 7 years. But, I wanted to leave that relationship so bad. My ideals of a progressive, bi-racial, brown & black, left wing, non-traditional-relationship bubble had been burst. We were no longer that. And, I began to wonder, had we ever been? Or had I been fooling myself all along?

More and more, I started to see I was aping the majority, meaning I was the majority, and his idea of marriage was traditional.

"You're taking my name," he said.

"Um, no I wasn't planning on it."

"Well, why did we get married then?"

He was clearly upset. I felt a lot of guilt. I had pursued the marriage more than he did.

"Okay, I will change my name."

I had let myself and my people down.

There were so many red flags that I chose to ignore. I will tell you why I ignored red flags and why we often do. I had to know. I had to know what I liked and did not like. I had to know who I truly was in my core. I had to learn from experience. Because I knew I liked men. And there was a part of me that wanted balance. I had spent 8 years with women, and for some reason I needed to be with this man.

People want us to heed advice, learn from their mistakes, and sometimes we can. We can learn from our elders, what we see on TV, and other times we must live it, despite all the cautionary tales, we must make our own mistakes.

After we got married, tradition, culture, and family were taking more of a front seat for him. Or maybe he was always like that, and I just never saw it. Maybe I chose to ignore it. Or maybe I just didn't understand it because I never bought in. And, although I looked straight, I had no idea what it meant to be a wife.

"I am a bartender, and my wife comes home later than me." He would say things like this to me often, letting me know I was a crappy "wife."

I was a party girl in his eyes, to his utter embarrassment. To be fair, I was also playing in a rock band, which I would later find out was also a problem.

And, coming of age in the LGBTQ community, as I had, was all about chosen family, meaning we were a lot of misfits, queers, many colors, coming together, and the nightclub and bar scene was often our home, a place where our chosen families could congregate.

Heterosexual people do not understand this. He certainly did not understand this.

There was no explaining this. To him, I was straight. I was a straight girl who stayed out late. Although I dated women when we met. He was outraged. I wanted the marriage, yet I had no idea how to be a wife. And then of course, true to toxic masculinity, my inability to be a "wife" must mean I was out there being unfaithful, and then his jealousy would take over.

"I mean, I don't even know who you are out with. Is it Tom, Dick, Larry or Mary?" He was accusing me of cheating.

There were other things that were wrong. For one, same-sex marriage wasn't even legal. Why would I marry when my same-sex cohorts couldn't? What kind of lesbian was I? Could I even call myself that anymore? I was back in the closet. I was the majority. And I was fucking that up, too. I didn't even know how to be a good wife. I was a shitty straight person.

When we met, he had been all on board for my lesbianism.

"It's like a breath of fresh air," he had said, and I felt so special, like I was somehow better than all those other women before me.

I would later learn that it is not uncommon for heterosexual men to like lesbian women. (How had I missed that one?) It also probably meant that I wasn't sleeping around with his male friends, or acquaintances, so it gave him the upper hand. I hadn't realized that I was inadvertently enabling his toxic masculinity, his desire to be special, territorial. Let's be clear, he didn't want a lesbian, he wanted a virgin. And, no actual virgin would want to have anything to do with a player, because that is what he was. However, a seasoned lesbian with an open sex positive lifestyle, well, was all too eager to say, "Let's do this."

*** NOTE: Virginity is a social construct, and most people who subscribe to this notion are in fact steeped in some religious upbringing which did not teach sex education, and instead leans on abstinence as a form of education, similar to the dark ages.)

He said, "Yea. You be you, I'll be me."

It sounded ideal.

And I fell for it.

All too eager.

It was everything BUT cool.

It wasn't long before I was lonely and wondering where he was all the time, wishing I had more of a social life. But, being kicked out of the Lesbian community when we started dating, I'd lost my social circle, my friends, my place in society. I couldn't just go to The Café anymore without being labeled a traitor: "Oh, she's dating a guy now." I could see them, hear them whispering about me. I could tell by the way they now avoided me. I could tell because I felt like I no longer belonged there. *TRAITOR* might as well have been tattooed on my forehead. I'm sure I horrified the fuck out of some and was a huge disappointment to others.

I understood it, too. I hated myself for it. How could I fight the patriarchy and simultaneously support it. I was a huge disappointment to the movement. And, to myself.

And yet there were actually quite a few "lesbians" who also dated men, too. For me, it was a wake-up call that we are multi-dimensional beings with the capacity to love and feel desire outside of what society was dictating for us. For me, it was a wake-up call that these political boundaries were too rigid.

Because right now I am regretting my choice.

Should I have rushed out of that situation, got a place of my own and went back to being a lonely lesbian? The me today says hell yes, you should have. What were you thinking? But I was already so lonely. And, I had been so lonely for the past few years. Lonely single. Lonely coupled. Lonely lesbian. Lonely person who wasn't pursuing art and the creative life I wanted. Lonely to the point I couldn't even create, even if I wanted to. Loneliness does that to you. It robs you of your resilience. There were so many things I wanted to do: travel, write, play music, live in big cities, but in my heart (or was it my head?) I knew I had to stick to something, and do it, instead of jumping from thing to thing. So, I chose to stick it out. Making rash decisions often just leads to more need for change, and ultimately makes it difficult to accomplish anything.

Even though those early days in San Francisco when he and I had just moved in together, in the dingy apartment in the Mission District, I wasn't accomplishing anything, I wasn't working towards anything, and he was out "seeing a man about a dog," which meant he was out with his guy friends smoking weed and felt like the most machismo thing in the world, I still decided to stick it out.

I didn't embrace queer politics enough and I blame myself because maybe there was a bisexual movement I could have gotten support from. But, as someone who had experienced so much oppression, I know this now, I didn't have the energy. I was frozen.

I couldn't get behind dyke politics 100% because I was sexually fluid, and my gender was fluid too. As much as I loved the politics and understood them (and wanted to fight for them) I was also drawn to the truth. My truth. I was bisexual, and suddenly I was having these strong urges to expand, to push at my edges and explore these other sides of myself, something I suddenly felt I could no longer do while being immersed in the lesbian community.

And, as painful and isolating as it was, I had to go figure this out for myself.

So, I did. I stayed in the most heteronormative, misogynistic, straight poop relationship ever. For 12 years.

What I learned is that sexuality is fluid. It's more fluid than this idea of homosexual versus heterosexual, it has layers upon layers. Everyone's expression is unique and no one version is correct, or alike for that matter.

For what it's worth, I now identify as a pansexual, non-monogamous, demi-sexual, semi-romantic. But it took a long time for me to embrace my intersections and to recognize that these intersections may and do shift.

I never questioned my straightness or my gayness. My ability to be sexually fluid would shift as I got older. Sometimes it was easier to connect with men, and I was attracted to men, so why not. Sometimes connecting with women was easier. But there was never a space where I felt safe saying I like men and women. I like the person. I like both. There was always so much judgment, so many questions. There still is.

What I did know was that I hated (still do) misogyny, the patriarchy, the toxic masculinity, men's inability to be emotionally intelligent (they don't have to be - and this is their privilege), men's lack of understanding or even sympathy around the female experience, homophobia, men's privilege which is best explained by this blanket entitlement men have around access and sex, and men's lack of awareness about the queer, femme experience in general.

I identify with the queer community, certainly as a political position.

And the political is personal, especially when you are a queer, woman of color. I wish I knew I had more choices. I wish I had the strength to create them.

When I started dating men, I lost all credibility in the queer world.

When you ape the majority, you reap the privileges of the heteronormative, cis gendered world. Even if you are bi, polyamorous, non-binary.

But me, I lost my voice.

Our society has passing standards, and most people, especially those who identify as queer or are marginalized, suffer from these passing standards because they make the rest of our dimensions invisible.

When I was dating women, I wasn't going around being super verbal or vocal about being queer, or bi, or lesbian, but I was attending events like Pride, frequenting gay bars, watching queer, LGBTQIA independent movies, and reading gay literature, so when I started dating men, I needed to be louder and prouder. But I didn't know where I could do that, or how.

"You date men now?"

The gay world rejected me, and ironically so did the straight world. Not in the ways you'd suspect. Of course, now I was legal to get married, to have joint bank accounts. I was getting passes left and right as a woman who was part of a heterosexual couple, but it was wrong. I was getting passes based on limited choices I'd made and how it looked on the outside, not based on who I really was. I was still oppressed, and it was killing me slowly.

Because let's be real. There's a truth we must talk about at some point, and that the reality is this competition, this territorial system stems from the patriarchy, from monogamy between women. Women have had to fight to stay alive. Their sisters are their greatest enemies, and it's the saddest thing in the world. When I entered the straight world, I wasn't entirely prepared for this.

Whatever your intersections you must see where they lie on the privilege continuum. For there are spaces for all of us and boxes we must all check.

I never was able to speak out about my bisexuality until much later and even now I still find this difficult. But I know that I must. I know that this is a normal expression of who I am. I know that in order to dismantle the long standing patriarchy, white supremacy, I must not only embrace but speak out not just about my sexuality, but about my skin color, my body type, the three main things that have oppressed me, while also embracing my privilege of growing up in an upper middle class society in a first world country with access to the best education, and all the resources afforded me to get ahead in this life. I must acknowledge all of it.

I have been on this journey for a while. And I am still on it. There are days when I will make mistakes, and there are days, oh so many days, that I will hide. This is hard and scary. And there are days I will show up.

I will keep going, as I know we have work to do. All I ask is that we be gentle with one another, try our best and stay the course.

www.ingramcontent.com/pod-product-compliance
Lightning Source LLC
Chambersburg PA
CBHW031600110426
42742CB00036B/573